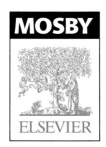

Nael E. A. Saad,
Instructor
Department of Rac   ar and
    Interventional R
Mallinckrodt Institu
Washington University School of Medicine
St. Louis, Missouri

D1028518

Suresh Vedantham, MD
Professor
Department of Radiology and Surgery
Mallinckrodt Institute of Radiology
Washington University School of Medicine
St. Louis, Missouri

Jennifer E. Gould, MD
Assistant Professor
Department of Radiology, Section of Vascular and
    Interventional Radiology
Mallinckrodt Institute of Radiology
Washington University School of Medicine
St. Louis, Missouri

CASE REVIEW

Vascular and Interventional Imaging

SECOND EDITION

CASE REVIEW SERIES

1600 John F. Kennedy Blvd.
Suite 1800
Philadelphia, PA 19103-2899

VASCULAR AND INTERVENTIONAL IMAGING, CASE REVIEW   ISBN-13: 978-0-323-05249-8
                                                     ISBN-10: 0-323-05249-5

NOTICE

Knowledge and best practice in this field are constantly changing. As new research and experience broaden our knowledge, changes in practice, treatment, and drug therapy may become necessary or appropriate. Readers are advised to check the most current information provided (i) on procedures featured; or (ii) by the manufacturer of each product to be administered, to verify the recommended dose or formula, the method and duration of administration, and contraindications. It is the responsibility of the practitioner, relying on their own experience and knowledge of the patient, to make diagnoses, to determine dosages and the best treatment for each individual patient, and to take all appropriate safety precautions. To the fullest extent of the law, neither the Publisher nor the Editors assume any liability for any injury and/or damage to persons or property arising out or related to any use of the material contained in this book.

Library of Congress Cataloging-in-Publication Data

Saad, Nael E. A.
  Vascular and interventional imaging : case review / Nael E. A.
Saad, Jennifer E. Gould, Suresh Vedantham. – 2nd ed.
     p. ; cm. – (Case review series)
  Rev. ed. of: Vascular & interventional imaging / Suresh Vedantham, Jennifer E. Gould.
2004.
  Cross referenced to: Vascular and interventional radiology : the requisites / John A.
Kaufman, Michael J. Lee. 2004.
  Includes bibliographical references and index.
  ISBN 978-0-323-05249-8 (alk. paper)
  1. Blood-vessels–Imaging–Case studies. 2.Blood-vessels–Interventional radiology–Case studies.
I. Gould, Jennifer E. II. Vedantham, Suresh. III. Vedantham, Suresh. Vascular & interventional
imaging. IV. Kaufman, John A. Vascular and interventional radiology. V. Title. VI. Series:
Case review series.
  [DNLM: 1. Vascular Diseases–radiography–Case Reports. 2. Vascular Diseases–radiography–
Problems and Exercises. 3. Radiography, Interventional–methods–Case Reports. 4. Radiography,
Interventional–methods–Problems and Exercises. WG 18.2 S111v 2010]
  RC691.6.I52V43 2010
  616.1'30754–dc22

                                                          2009014660

Acquisitions Editor: Rebecca Gaertner
Developmental Editor: Colleen McGonigal
Project Manager: Nayagi Athmanathan
Design Direction: Steven Stave

Printed in the United States of America
Last digit is the print number: 9 8 7 6 5 4 3 2 1

For my parents and my brother Wael
NS

For my parents, Vasanth, Tanya, and Shrey
SV

For my parents, my husband Jim, and our daughter Ava.
JG

I have been very gratified by the popularity and positive feedback that the authors of the Case Review Series have received upon the publication of the first edition of their volumes. Reviews in journals and word-of-mouth comments have been uniformly favorable. The authors have done an outstanding job in filling the niche of an affordable, easy-reading, case-based learning tool that supplements the material in *THE REQUISITES* series. I have been told by residents, fellows, and practicing radiologists that the Case Review Series books are the ideal means for studying for oral Boards and subspecialty certification tests.

It was recognized that while some students learn best in a non-interactive study-book mode, others need the anxiety or excitement of being quizzed, being put on the hot seat. The format that was selected for the Case Review Series, i.e., showing a limited number of images needed to construct a differential diagnosis and asking a few clinical and imaging questions was designed to simulate the Boards experience (the only difference is that the Case Review books provide the correct answer and immediate feedback). Cases are scaled from relatively easy to very hard to test the limit of the reader's knowledge. In addition, a brief authors' commentary, a link back to *THE REQUISITES* volume, and an up-to-date reference in the literature are provided.

Because of the popularity of the series, we have been rolling out the second editions of the Case Review Series volumes. The expectation is that the second editions will bring the content up to the current knowledge limits of the field, introduce new modalities and new techniques, and provide new and even more graphic examples of pathology.

This volume of the Case Review Series, *Vascular and Interventional Imaging*, authored by Nael Saad, Suresh Vedantham, and Jennifer Gould, reflects the unique philosophy of clinical care that now permeates the field of Interventional Radiology (IR) (and to some extent Breast Imaging). The physicians in IR are the nexus to surgeons, internists, hospitalists, and radiologists. They take care of the whole patient—inpatient and outpatient, preoperatively, intraoperatively, and postoperatively. The authors have provided a wonderful set of cases that not only are applicable as a review of the practice for Boards and to enhance one's knowledge base. The cases also bring to fore the need for clinical judgment and compassion when practicing in this unique field. The latest edition also provides more evidence-based data on outcomes of existing and newly developed interventional techniques.

I am pleased to present for your eminent pleasure *Vascular and Interventional Imaging*, second edition of the Case Review Series by Drs. Saad, Vedantham, and Gould, joining the previous second editions of Head and Neck Imaging by David M. Yousem and Carol Motta; *Genitourinary Imaging* by Ronald J. Zagoria, William W. Mayo-Smith, and Julia R. Fielding; *Obstetric and Gynecologic Ultrasound* by Karen L. Reuter and T. Kemi Babagbemi; *General and Vascular Ultrasound* by William D. Middleton; *Spine Imaging* by Brian C. Bowen, Alfonso Rivera, and Efrat Saraf-Lavi; *Musculoskeletal Imaging* by Joseph S. Yu; *Gastrointestinal Imaging* by Robert D. Halpert; *Brain Imaging* by Laurie Loevner; and *Emergency Radiology* by Stuart E. Mirvis, Kathirkamanathan Shanmuganathan, Lisa A. Miller, and Clint W. Sliker.

David M. Yousem, MD, MBA

The Case Review Series provides an interactive case review format which challenges the reader to demonstrate both interpretive accuracy and an understanding of the clinical relevance of imaging findings. As such, it could not be better suited to address the unique and dynamic challenges associated with learning Interventional Radiology. Optimizing subspecialty Board examination preparation is a primary goal of *Vascular and Interventional Imaging*; however, two additional goals are central to our conception of the book's value.

First, we showcase numerous diagnostic and therapeutic procedures which are performed by the modern interventional radiologist. The image of Interventional Radiology held by a typical Radiology trainee often reflects only those few case types to which he/she has been exposed. However, the reader of this book will discover cases involving a broad range of arterial, venous, and non-vascular procedures, and will observe how they impact upon many disease processes. Included in the Challenge section are cases involving several very new procedures which define the outer edge of Interventional Radiology knowledge in 2009. Our sincere hope is that the "impressive" display of this broad spectrum will stimulate trainees to explore the possibilities of subspecializing in this exciting field.

Second, the reader will notice that a significant amount of presented material pertains to the proper *clinical evaluation* and *treatment* of patients. In our view, this material is critical in enabling the reader to develop and convey (to referring physician, colleague, and board examiner alike) a fundamentally mature procedure-related clinical judgment level which every radiologist should possess. The speed with which interventionalists are adopting the practice patterns and responsibilities of our clinical colleagues in other disciplines is accelerating, and only a superb grounding in clinical and therapeutic principles will enable the modern trainee to keep pace.

In the second edition, we have added a few procedures that have developed and gained favor in the field of modern Interventional Radiology. Additionally, we have updated existing case discussions to reflect the current data in the literature.

We certainly hope that *Vascular and Interventional Imaging* will prove to be a valuable resource for all current practitioners and trainees in General and Interventional Radiology.

Nael Saad, MB, BCh
Suresh Vedantham, MD
Jennifer Gould, MD

We sincerely thank and acknowledge the many contributions of our Interventional Radiology colleagues. Specifically, we are indebted to Drs. Daniel Brown, Thomas Vesely, James Duncan, David Hovsepian, Michael Darcy, Sailendra Naidu, and Daniel Picus for being exceedingly generous in sharing the clinical gems hidden in their personal teaching files. Many thanks also go to Simone Werner for her diligent effort in helping with the completion of this work, to Rebecca Gaertner at Elsevier, and to Series editor Dr. David Yousem for his vision, guidance, and encouragement, and for the wonderful opportunity he has given us.

Opening Round

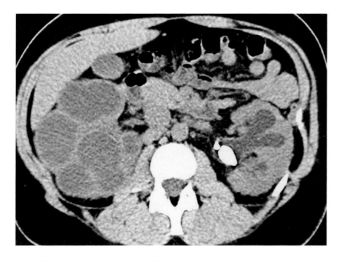 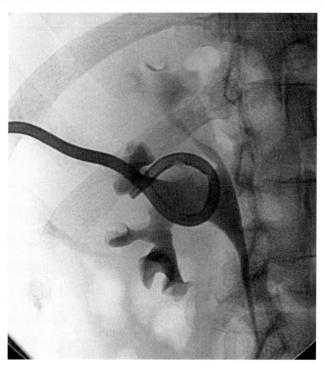

1. What treatment would you recommend for this 32-year-old woman with fever, flank pain, leukocytosis, and urinalysis consistent with urinary tract infection?

2. Unilateral or bilateral?

3. When should this procedure be performed?

4. What is the most common cause of this diagnosis?

Pyonephrosis

1. Percutaneous nephrostomy tube insertion.

2. Bilateral.

3. Urgently.

4. Urinary tract stones.

Reference

Watson RA, Esposito M, Richter F. Percutaneous nephrostomy as adjunct management in advanced upper urinary tract infection. *Urology.* 1999;54:234-239.

Cross-Reference

Vascular and Interventional Radiology: THE REQUISITES, pp 608-615.

Comment

The CT examination demonstrates bilateral hydronephrosis. Although percutaneous nephrostomy tubes can be inserted electively for relief of urinary obstruction, clinical signs of infection are concerning for pyonephrosis: infected urine within the obstructed urinary collecting system. Such patients are at risk for sepsis, and percutaneous nephrostomy should be performed urgently. In the patient who already exhibits signs of sepsis, percutaneous nephrostomy can be life-saving and must be performed emergently.

Percutaneous nephrostomy tubes can be placed using a variety of imaging guidance techniques. If contrast material is already present from an existing study or if an existing ureteral stent or radiopaque renal calculus is present, then fluoroscopic guidance alone may be sufficient. Otherwise, ultrasound- or CT-guided puncture of a posterior calyx can be performed (one-pass method). Alternatively, if a dilated posterior calyx is not clearly visible, then the renal pelvis can be punctured with a 22-gauge needle. A small amount of contrast and air are injected to opacify a posterior calyx, which is then definitively punctured using an 18-gauge needle under fluoroscopic guidance (two-pass method).

Although any cause of urinary tract obstruction can lead to hydronephrosis or pyonephrosis, more than 50% of cases result from urinary tract calculi. Another common cause is ureteral compression by a pelvic mass lesion. Definitive removal of the obstructing agent should be deferred to a time when the patient's infection has resolved, because excessive manipulation can precipitate sepsis.

Notes

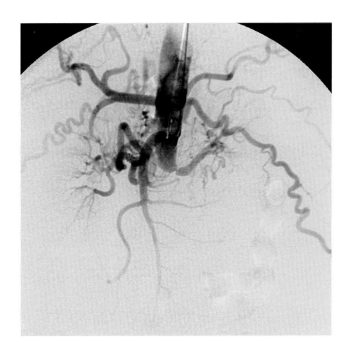

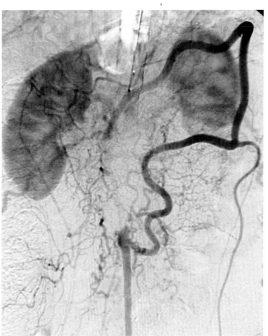

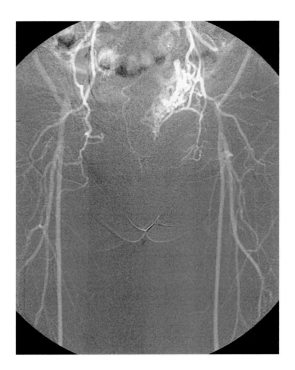

1. What abnormality is seen in the first image?

2. What is the most likely etiology?

3. Would you describe this as an acute event or a chronic event?

4. How is blood reaching the lower extremities in this patient?

Abdominal Aortic Occlusion
(Leriche's Syndrome)

1. Occlusion of the infrarenal abdominal aorta with enlarged lumbar collaterals.

2. Atherosclerosis.

3. This most likely represents thrombosis at the site of a chronic stenosis.

4. Superior mesenteric artery to inferior mesenteric artery via an enlarged marginal artery of Drummond (second image), to the internal iliac arterial system and finally to the common femoral arteries.

Reference

Bosch JL, Huninck MC. Meta-analysis of the results of percutaneous transluminal angioplasty and stent placement for aorto-iliac occlusive disease. *Radiology.* 1997;204:87-96.

Cross-Reference

Vascular and Interventional Radiology: THE REQUI-SITES, pp 261-270.

Comment

Occlusion of the abdominal aorta can result from a variety of causes including trauma, thromboembolism, or iatrogenic dissection. In this case, thrombosis is superimposed on chronic atherosclerotic stenosis, a condition known as *Leriche's syndrome.* In these patients, symptoms of ischemia might not appear until occlusion is imminent, and some patients present after the vessel has occluded. The classic symptoms of Leriche's syndrome are seen in men and include hip and buttock claudication, absent femoral pulses, impotence (due to limitation of blood flow into the internal iliac artery territories), and cool lower extremities.

The slow progression of the atherosclerotic occlusion allows the development of large intercostal, lumbar and epigastric collaterals that provide flow to the iliac arteries and lower-extremity vessels. The treatment of choice for Leriche's syndrome is surgical bypass graft placement; in this case, an aorto-bifemoral graft would be appropriate. In patients who are not surgical candidates, endoluminal recanalization and stenting of the occluded aorta and iliac arteries can be performed.

Notes

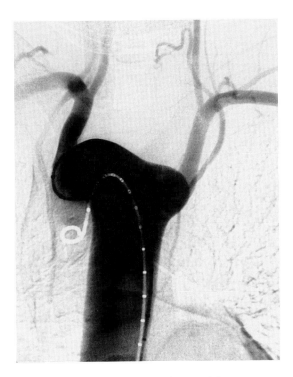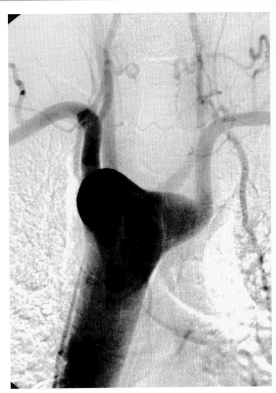

1. What is the most likely diagnosis?

2. Does this represent a vascular ring?

3. Does this finding usually indicate the presence of congenital heart disease?

4. Does this finding typically cause airway compression?

Variant Anatomy: Right-Sided Aortic Arch

1. Right aortic arch with aberrant left subclavian artery.

2. Yes.

3. No.

4. No.

References

Franquet T, Erasmus JJ, Gimenez A. The retrotracheal space: Normal anatomic and pathologic appearances. *Radiographics.* 2002;22:S231-S246.

Donnelly LF, Fleck RJ, Pacharn P, et al. Aberrant subclavian arteries: Cross-sectional imaging findings in infants and children referred for evaluation of extrinsic airway compression. *Am J Roentgenol.* 2002;178: 1269-1274.

Cross-Reference

Vascular and Interventional Radiology: THE REQUISITES, pp 219-222.

Comment

A right-sided aortic arch with aberrant left subclavian artery occurs in 0.05% to 0.10% of the population. The aortic arch passes over the right mainstem bronchus and descends to the right of the esophagus and trachea. The left subclavian artery arises as the last branch, often from a diverticulum of Kommerell, as in this case, and passes behind the trachea and esophagus to supply the left arm. Symptoms of respiratory and esophageal compression are seen in only 5%. Only 10% of patients have associated congenital heart disease, most commonly tetralogy of Fallot.

Right aortic arch can also be seen with mirror-image branching. In this situation, the aortic branch vessels in order are the left brachiocephalic artery, right common carotid artery, and right subclavian artery. More than 98% of these patients have cyanotic congenital heart disease, most commonly tetralogy of Fallot.

Notes

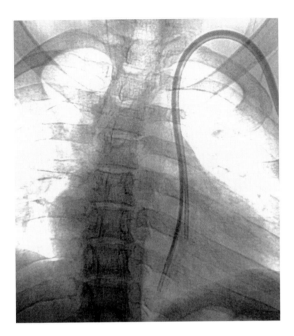 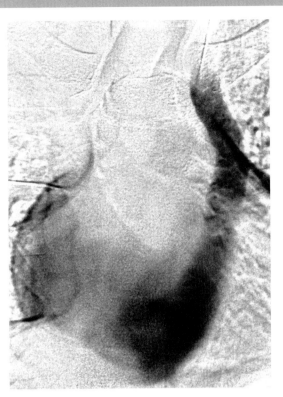

1. What vessel does this dialysis catheter traverse just before reaching the heart?

2. How does blood typically reach the right atrium in this anatomic variant?

3. Is there an association with congenital heart disease?

4. What anatomic variant is in the differential diagnosis?

C A S E 4

Variant Anatomy: Left Superior Vena Cava

1. Left superior vena cava.

2. Via the coronary sinus.

3. Yes.

4. Duplicated superior vena cava.

Reference

Minniti S, Visentini S, Procacci C. Congenital anomalies of the venae cavae: Embryological origin, imaging features and report of three new variants. *Eur Radiol.* 2002;12:2040-2055.

Cross-Reference

Vascular and Interventional Radiology: THE REQUISITES, p 165.

Comment

A left superior vena cava results from persistence of the left anterior cardinal vein. This usually occurs in association with congenital heart disease, although it occurs rarely as an isolated abnormality associated with situs inversus. Typically, the left superior vena cava drains to the right atrium via the coronary sinus, but occasionally it drains directly into the left atrium.

Duplication of the superior vena cava is more common and is even more often associated with congenital heart disease. It can be associated with anomalous pulmonary venous return. Similar to the isolated left superior vena cava, the left moiety typically drains into the coronary sinus.

Notes

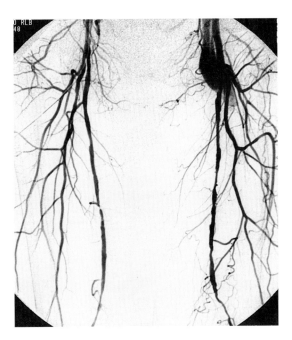 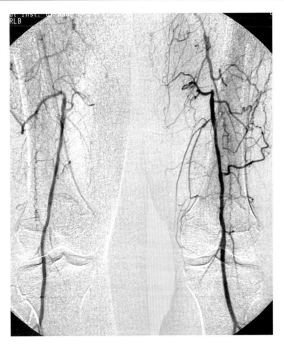

1. What type of examination is depicted above and how was it performed?

2. What is the primary abnormality in the right leg?

3. What surgical treatment can be used for this problem?

4. Would endovascular stent placement be a good alternative to surgery?

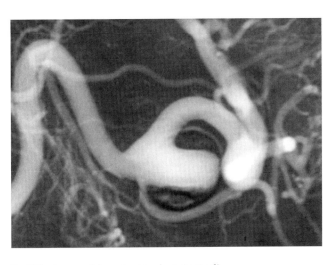 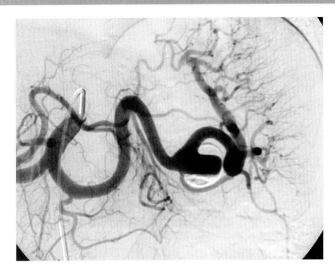

1. What vessel is selectively injected?

2. What is the abnormality?

3. When is treatment recommended?

4. What treatment methods can be used?

CASE 5

Occluded Superficial Femoral Artery

1. Bilateral lower-extremity digital subtraction arteriogram. A catheter has been placed via the right common femoral artery (CFA) into the aorta or into the right iliac artery.

2. Right superficial femoral artery (SFA) occlusion with popliteal reconstitution.

3. Femoropopliteal bypass graft placement.

4. Self-expanding nitinol stents may be used for treating this condition, but they should be reserved for patients who are not candidates for surgery.

Reference

Hunink M, Wong J, Donaldson, et al. Revascularization for femoropopliteal disease: A decision and cost-effectiveness analysis. *JAMA*. 1995;274:165-171.

Cross-Reference

Vascular and Interventional Radiology: THE REQUISITES, pp 419-428.

Comment

The SFA represents an extremely common site of atherosclerotic disease. Stenotic lesions in this vessel are most commonly observed at the level of the adductor (Hunter's) canal. These lesions are a common cause of calf claudication and can contribute (in the presence of other lesions) to rest pain and limb-threatening ischemia. Progressive SFA stenosis often leads to complete SFA occlusion.

When describing a lesion in the SFA, several observations are important to make: (1) The status of the ipsilateral CFA is important because this vessel nearly always represents the source vessel for a therapeutic bypass graft; (2) The point at which the distal circulation reconstitutes, as well as its continuity with pedal flow, determines the distal anastomotic site of the bypass graft; (3) The status of the ipsilateral profunda femoral artery often determines the clinical status of the limb, because this vessel provides the source for the collaterals that reconstitute the distal circulation.

The standard treatment of isolated SFA occlusion with popliteal reconstitution is femoropopliteal bypass graft placement. This procedure has a 5-year patency of 50% to 80%, depending on whether the distal anastomosis is placed above or below the knee and depending on the number and quality of patent runoff vessels. Catheter-directed thrombolysis with subsequent angioplasty and stenting can be used to recanalize native SFA occlusions, but patency rates following this procedure are less than those of surgical therapy.

CASE 6

Splenic Artery Aneurysm

1. Celiac artery.

2. Splenic artery aneurysm.

3. Treatment is recommended when the aneurysm is large (>2.5 cm), symptomatic, or rapidly expanding and in women who are or might become pregnant.

4. Transcatheter embolization (preferred in most cases) or surgical resection.

Reference

Stanley JC. Mesenteric arterial occlusive and aneurysmal disease. *Cardiol Clin*. 2002;20:611-622.

Cross-Reference

Vascular and Interventional Radiology: THE REQUISITES, pp 314-317.

Comment

The splenic artery is the most common site of visceral artery aneurysms, followed by the hepatic artery. Splenic artery aneurysms are more common in women than men. The most common etiology is medial degeneration with superimposed atherosclerosis. There appears to be some relationship to pregnancy because the majority of women who have splenic artery aneurysms have had at least two pregnancies, and pregnancy is associated with an increased risk of rupture. Other causes include trauma, pancreatitis, infection, congenital portal hypertension, collagen vascular disease, hypersplenism, fibromuscular dysplasia, and vasculitis.

Many aneurysms are discovered incidentally on cross-sectional imaging. The main risk is aneurysm rupture, which carries a high mortality. These patients typically present with abdominal pain and/or hypotension. Nevertheless, less than 10% of aneurysms rupture, and the majority of ruptures are associated with pregnancy. Therefore, treatment is not recommended for all unruptured aneurysms.

Treatment is directed at eliminating flow into the aneurysm sac. Transcatheter embolization is the preferred treatment, and coils are the most commonly used agent. It is important to embolize from distal to proximal across the aneurysm neck to prevent retrograde flow into the aneurysm from collateral vessels filling the distal splenic artery. Splenic infarction or abscess formation is rare owing to collateral flow to the spleen. Splenic artery aneurysms can be treated surgically by removing the spleen and aneurysm or by ligating the artery proximal and distal to the aneurysm.

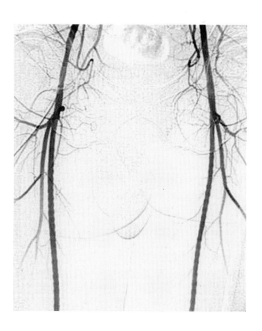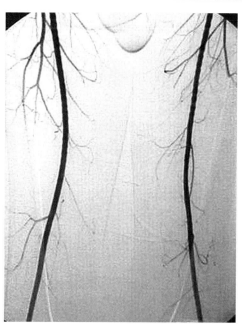

1. What is the main angiographic finding?

2. Is this pathologic?

3. What vascular beds most commonly demonstrate this finding?

4. What is the likely explanation?

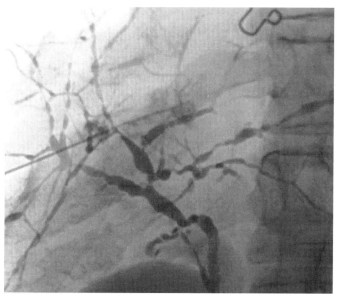

Courtesy of Dr. Daniel Brown.

1. What is the likely diagnosis?

2. Is this disorder more common in men or women?

3. Name three conditions that this disorder can be associated with.

4. Name three long-term complications of this disorder.

CASE 7

Normal Finding: Standing Waves

1. A regular corrugated appearance of the arteries, known as *standing waves*.

2. No.

3. The extremity arteries and mesenteric vessels.

4. Flow and pressure changes during contrast injection into a high-resistance vascular bed.

Reference

Reuter SR, Redman HC, Cho KJ. Vascular diseases. In: *Gastrointestinal Angiography*. 3rd ed. Philadelphia: Saunders; 1986:120-121.

Cross-Reference

Vascular and Interventional Radiology: THE REQUISITES, pp 18-22.

Comment

Standing waves are occasionally observed during arteriography of the extremities or mesenteric vessels. Appearing as regular alternating areas of constriction, they likely result from focal, circular vasoconstriction. Various hypotheses exist to explain this benign finding. All center on changes in flow and pressure resulting from injection of contrast media.

CASE 8

Sclerosing Cholangitis

1. Sclerosing cholangitis.

2. Men (70% of cases).

3. Inflammatory bowel disease, pancreatitis, mediastinal or retroperitoneal fibrosis.

4. Acute cholangitis episodes, biliary cirrhosis, cholangiocarcinoma.

Reference

Bader TR, Beavers KL, Semelka RC. MR imaging features of primary sclerosing cholangitis: Patterns of cirrhosis in relationship to clinical severity of disease. *Radiology*. 2003;226:675-685.

Cross-Reference

Vascular and Interventional Radiology: THE REQUISITES, pp 580-584.

Comment

Sclerosing cholangitis is an insidious progressive disease in which chronic inflammation and obliterative fibrosis affect the intrahepatic and extrahepatic biliary ductal system. Patients often present with chronic or intermittent obstructive jaundice, abdominal pain, fatigue, and/ or fever. The hallmark cholangiographic findings of sclerosing cholangitis include multifocal strictures, saccular outpouchings and areas of dilation, a beaded appearance of the biliary ductal system, and/or a pruned-tree appearance of the biliary system. The common bile duct is almost always involved. The differential diagnosis of these findings includes multifocal cholangiocarcinoma and primary biliary cirrhosis.

Sclerosing cholangitis can occur as a primary idiopathic disorder or in association with other inflammatory conditions, including ulcerative colitis, Crohn's disease, pancreatitis, retroperitoneal fibrosis, or mediastinal fibrosis. The dreaded long-term sequelae of this disorder are biliary cirrhosis with portal hypertension, and cholangiocarcinoma.

Medical management of primary sclerosing cholangitis is not particularly effective. Percutaneous biliary drainage or hepaticojejunostomy can provide palliation to carefully selected patients with appropriate anatomy, but the only truly effective treatment for this disorder is liver transplantation.

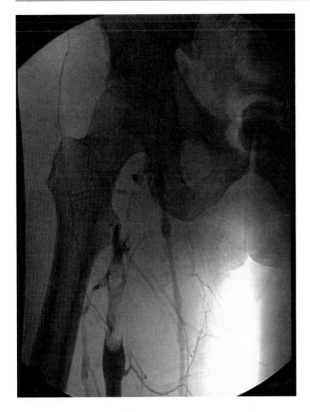

1. What type of study has been performed?

2. What is the diagnosis?

3. How long have the patient's symptoms likely been present?

4. What treatment options might be considered?

C A S E 9

Acute Deep Vein Thrombosis

1. Lower-extremity venogram.

2. Acute femoral deep vein thrombosis (DVT).

3. Less than 2 weeks.

4. Anticoagulation is the traditional standard of care. Selected patients with acute iliofemoral DVT may be treated with catheter-directed thrombolysis or surgical thrombectomy. Elastic compression stockings should be worn for at least 2 years to prevent post-thrombotic syndrome. Patients who have contraindications to anticoagulation should undergo filter placement in the inferior vena cava for prophylaxis of pulmonary embolism.

Reference

Vedantham S, Millward SF, Cardella JF, et al. Society of Interventional Radiology: Society of Interventional Radiology position statement. Treatment of acute iliofemoral deep vein thrombosis with use of adjunctive catheter-directed intrathrombus thrombolysis. *J Vasc Interv Radiol.* 2006;17(4):613-616.

Cross-Reference

Vascular and Interventional Radiology: THE REQUISITES, pp 452-457.

Comment

Lower-extremity DVT is a significant cause of morbidity and long-term disability. The immediate complications of DVT can include pulmonary embolism and limb-threatening phlegmasia. In the long term, a large fraction of DVT patients experience post-thrombotic symptoms, which include limb heaviness and aching, ambulatory edema, venous claudication, and lower extremity ulcerations.

The diagnosis of DVT in the femoropopliteal veins can be made with high accuracy using duplex ultrasound. In contrast, lower-extremity venography, the gold standard for the diagnosis of DVT, is only infrequently required for diagnosis. Venography is more often used to evaluate for DVT in the iliac venous system, which is often not well visualized by ultrasound. Venographic findings of acute (< 2 weeks) DVT typically include globular filling defects within a vein, abrupt occlusion of the vein, and/or dilation of the distal venous system. In this case, globular elongated filling defects are present within the femoral vein.

The standard treatment for patients with DVT is anticoagulation using low-molecular-weight or unfractionated heparin followed by coumadin for at least 3 months in most instances.

Patients with iliofemoral DVT have a particularly high risk of developing a severe form of post-thrombotic syndrome. For this reason, selected patients with acute iliofemoral DVT are treated with catheter-directed thrombolysis or surgical venous thrombectomy.

Notes

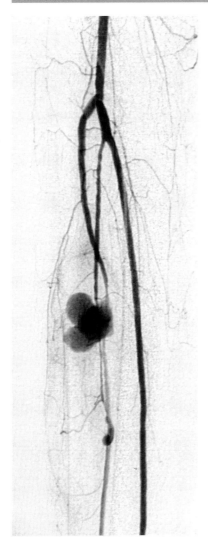

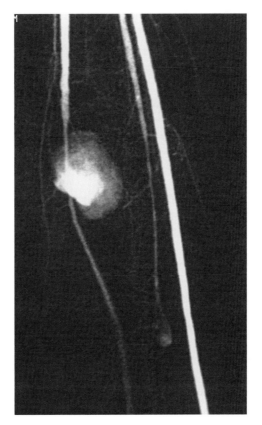

1. What abnormality is present?

2. What is the likely etiology of this abnormality?

3. How can patients with this problem be treated?

4. What imaging modality is best used for follow-up after treatment?

Tibial Artery Pseudoaneurysm

1. Large saccular pseudoaneurysm of the anterior tibial artery.

2. Trauma, iatrogenic vascular injury, or infection.

3. Surgical repair of the vessel is usually employed. In select cases where the vessel does not provide significant arterial supply to the foot, angiographic embolization may be performed.

4. Duplex ultrasound.

Reference

Wolford H, Peterson SL, Ray C, et al. Delayed arteriovenous fistula and pseudoaneurysm after an open tibial fracture successfully managed with selective angiographic embolization. *J Trauma*. 2001;51:781-783.

Cross-Reference

Vascular and Interventional Radiology: THE REQUISITES, pp 437-439.

Comment

Peripheral pseudoaneurysms of medium-sized vessels most commonly occur in the setting of trauma. In this case, the trauma was probably caused by Fogarty catheter embolectomy of the tibial arteries following revision of a thrombosed femoropopliteal bypass graft (not shown). Although mycotic aneurysm is rare, the possibility should be considered when saccular or irregular aneurysms are seen in the periphery.

Although duplex ultrasound can diagnose and localize the pseudoaneurysm, arteriography is important in planning appropriate therapy. It is important to determine the exact location of the entry into the pseudoaneurysm and to completely evaluate the arterial runoff to the extremity. When the injured vessel still makes a significant contribution to perfusion of the lower extremity, surgical repair of the vessel or ligation with distal bypass is clearly indicated. In select instances when this is not the case, arterial embolization may be undertaken. In this instance, it is important to place coils within the artery both proximal and distal to the origin of the pseudoaneurysm.

Notes

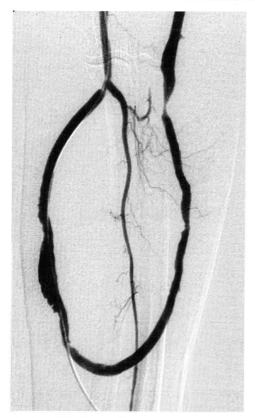

Courtesy of Dr. Thomas Vesely.

1. What type of examination is depicted?

2. What symptoms are likely to be present?

3. What abnormality is seen on the image?

4. How might this problem be treated?

Dialysis Graft Stenoses

1. Dialysis fistulogram.

2. Low flows or high recirculation during dialysis.

3. Three stenoses are present: a tight stenosis at the venous anastomosis of the graft and two mild stenoses within the graft.

4. Angioplasty of the stenoses, or surgical graft revision.

Reference

National Kidney Foundation. Guidelines for vascular access. In *Kidney Disease Outcomes Quality Initiative Clinical Practice Guidelines*. New York: National Kidney Foundation; 2000.

Cross-Reference

Vascular and Interventional Radiology: THE REQUISITES, pp 184-191.

Comment

Hemodialysis can be performed from a variety of access routes: (1) A native fistula can be created between an extremity artery—usually a radial artery or brachial artery—and an adjacent vein; (2) A prosthetic graft—usually polytetrafluoroethylene—can be placed to attach a parent artery to an outflow vein; (3) A dialysis access catheter may be placed from a suitable central vein, preferably an internal jugular vein.

When a native fistula or prosthetic graft is used, suboptimal dialysis can occur due to formation of stenotic lesions somewhere in the vascular access circuit. The venous anastomosis of the graft is by far the most common site of stenosis in patients with prosthetic grafts, as in this case. However, suboptimal dialysis can also result from flow-limiting stenoses within the graft, within the outflow veins draining the graft, within the central venous system, at the arterial anastomosis, or even in the parent artery. Such lesions, in addition to causing suboptimal dialysis, ultimately lead to graft thrombosis in the majority of cases.

Improved duration of graft patency and improved dialysis quality can be achieved via successful treatment of stenotic lesions. This can be achieved surgically or via percutaneous transluminal angioplasty. The mean graft patency following angioplasty of a venous stenosis of a patent graft is approximately 6 months, but repeat angioplasty can often delay graft replacement for several years.

Notes

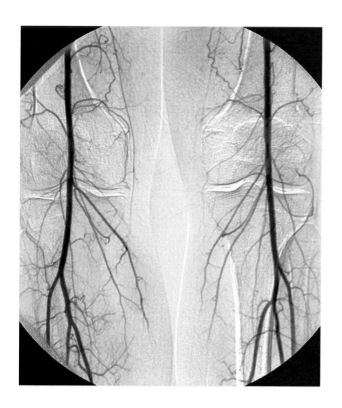

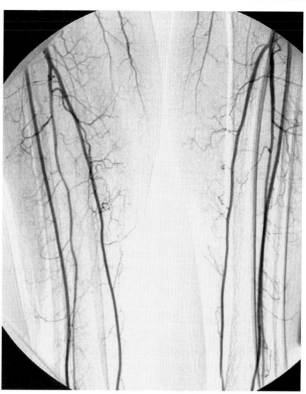

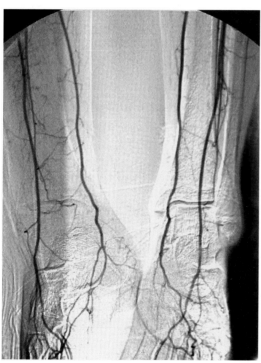

1. On an anteroposterior view of an angiogram, name the three tibial runoff arteries from lateral to medial.

2. Do most patients have a true trifurcation of the popliteal artery?

3. Which vessel continues into the foot as the dorsalis pedis artery?

4. Which vessel normally terminates above the ankle level?

Normal Tibial Artery Anatomy

1. Anterior tibial artery, peroneal artery, and posterior tibial artery.

2. No.

3. Anterior tibial artery.

4. Peroneal artery.

Reference

Toussarkissian B, Mejia A, Smilanich RP. Noninvasive localization of infrainguinal arterial occlusive disease in diabetics. *Ann Vasc Surg*. 2001;13:714-721.

Cross-Reference

Vascular and Interventional Radiology: THE REQUISITES, pp 407-411.

Comment

The popliteal artery begins distal to the adductor canal and passes through the popliteal fossa between the heads of the gastrocnemius muscle. At its terminal aspect it typically bifurcates into the anterior tibial artery and tibioperoneal trunk. After 2 to 3 cm, the tibioperoneal trunk in turn bifurcates into the peroneal and posterior tibial arteries. A true trifurcation of the popliteal artery is only present in a minority of patients.

In the normal patient, the anterior tibial artery continues across the ankle as the dorsalis pedis artery; the posterior tibial artery passes behind the medial malleolus into the foot, where it divides into the lateral and medial plantar arteries. These vessels then anastomose through dorsal and plantar arches within the foot. The peroneal artery runs in the interosseous membrane and typically gives off terminal branches proximal to the ankle that anastomose with branches from the posterior tibial artery and anterior tibial artery.

Notes

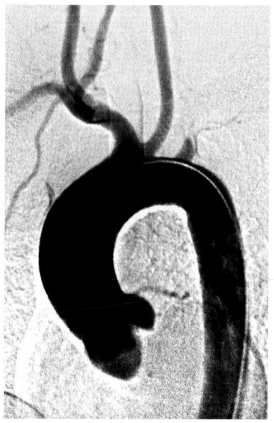

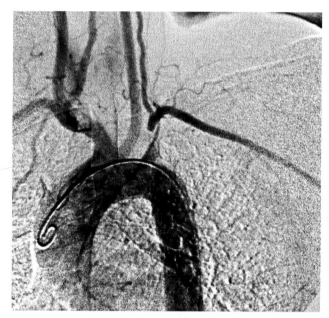

Courtesy of Dr. Daniel Brown.

Courtesy of Dr. Daniel Brown.

1. What angiographic abnormality is depicted?

2. What symptoms are likely being experienced by the patient?

3. Does this abnormality occur more commonly on the left or the right?

4. What is the most common etiology of this abnormality?

Subclavian Steal Syndrome

1. Subclavian steal syndrome.

2. Symptoms of vertebrobasilar insufficiency or, less likely, symptoms of brachial insufficiency.

3. Left (3:1 ratio).

4. Atherosclerosis.

Reference

Taylor CL, Selman WR, Ratcheson RA. Steal affecting the central nervous system. *Neurosurgery*. 2002;50: 679-688.

Cross-Reference

Vascular and Interventional Radiology: THE REQUI-SITES, pp 149-151.

Comment

Subclavian steal syndrome can occur due to stenosis or occlusion of the proximal segment of the subclavian artery. Most commonly, this lesion causes signs of vertebrobasilar insufficiency, including syncopal or near-syncopal episodes initiated by exercising the ipsilateral arm, headaches, nausea, vertigo, and other neurological symptoms. In a minority of patients, signs of brachial insufficiency are present, including upper-extremity pain, paresthesias, coolness, weakness, or fingertip necrosis.

The diagnosis is often suspected based on the clinical history and the physical finding of diminished pulse and/or diminished systolic blood pressure in the affected limb. Duplex ultrasound often demonstrates reversal of vertebral artery flow. The classic angiographic features of this diagnosis are the presence of stenosis or occlusion of the subclavian artery proximal to the vertebral artery origin, with retrograde flow down the vertebral artery seen later in the angiographic run. The lesion can be treated with either surgical bypass or angioplasty.

Notes

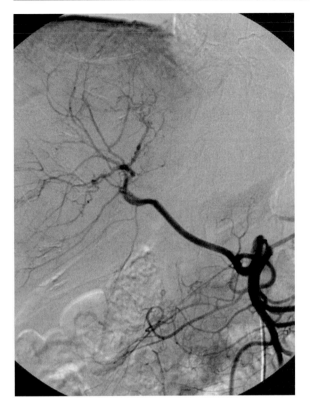 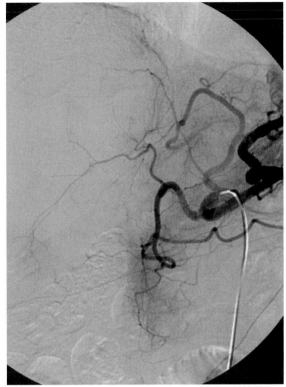

1. What anatomic variant is depicted in the first image?

2. Where does this vessel arise from?

3. What anatomic variants are depicted in the second image?

4. Where do these vessels arise from?

Variant Anatomy: Replaced Hepatic Arteries

1. Replaced right hepatic artery.

2. Superior mesenteric artery.

3. Replaced left hepatic artery and middle hepatic artery.

4. Left gastric artery and common hepatic artery.

Reference

Covey AM, Brody LA, Maluccio MA, et al. Variant hepatic arterial anatomy revisited: Digital subtraction angiography performed in 600 patients. *Radiology*. 2002; 224:542-547.

Cross-Reference

Vascular and Interventional Radiology: THE REQUISITES, pp 286-292.

Comment

It is important to recognize the common variants in the arterial supply to the liver. Vessels can be *replaced* or *accessory*, but vessels supplying the liver are typically not redundant. A *replaced* artery exists when the vessel supplying an entire hepatic lobe arises aberrantly. An *accessory* artery exists when a portion of a hepatic lobe is supplied by a vessel of normal origin but an additional vessel of aberrant origin also supplies a portion of the lobe.

Estimates vary, but approximately 15% to 25% of people have an accessory or replaced left hepatic artery arising from the left gastric artery. When it is difficult to determine whether left hepatic branches are arising from the left gastric artery, steep left anterior oblique and lateral views can help to separate hepatic branches (which run anteriorly to the left liver lobe) and gastric fundal branches.

Approximately 15% to 20% of people have an accessory or replaced right hepatic artery arising from the superior mesenteric artery. The replaced hepatic artery is almost invariably the first branch from the superior mesenteric artery in such cases. Additional rare variants have been described in which the entire hepatic arterial supply is derived from the superior mesenteric artery or aorta.

Notes

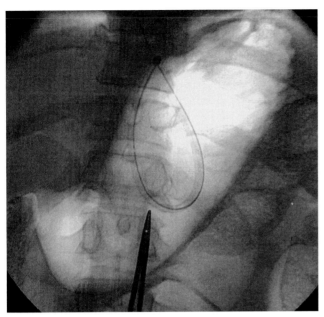

Courtesy of Dr. Daniel Brown.

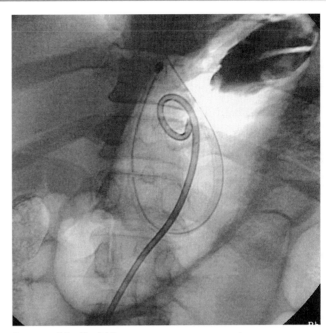

Courtesy of Dr. Daniel Brown.

1. What procedure has been performed?

2. Is general anesthesia required for this procedure?

3. Name two major complications of this procedure.

4. After the catheter is placed, what is the earliest time it can be removed?

Percutaneous Gastrostomy Placement

1. Percutaneous gastrostomy tube placement.

2. No.

3. Peritonitis and hemorrhage.

4. One month; a mature transperitoneal tract must be present.

Reference

Laasch HU, Wilbraham L, Bullen K. Gastrostomy insertion: Comparing the options—PEG, RIG or PIG? *Clin Radiol.* 2003;58:398-405.

Cross-Reference

Vascular and Interventional Radiology: THE REQUISITES, pp 521-532.

Comment

Percutaneous gastrostomy tube (G-tube) placement is performed for nutritional support in patients with inadequate oral intake or for gastric decompression in patients with chronic obstruction of the small bowel. Advantages of percutaneous G-tube placement over surgical placement include elimination of general anesthesia and its associated morbidity. Endoscopic placement has a higher incidence of aspiration and wound infection.

The basic method of G-tube placement involves the following steps: (1) The stomach is insufflated with air through a nasogastric tube; (2) Fluoroscopic confirmation of a safe access window into the stomach is confirmed, with careful attention to avoiding transcolonic or transhepatic puncture; (3) Percutaneous gastropexy may be performed via insertion of two to four metallic T-fasteners, which bring the anterior gastric wall up to the anterior abdominal wall. This is done routinely in some centers and selectively in others. Selected patients include those with ascites and patients who have diminished ability to form a secure transperitoneal tract around the catheter (e.g., patients receiving steroids); (4) A needle is placed in the gastric body, and contrast is injected to confirm intragastric positioning; (5) Over a guidewire, the tract is enlarged using sequential dilators; (6) The gastrostomy catheter is positioned in the stomach and contrast is injected to confirm adequate positioning.

Complications of percutaneous G-tube placement can include peritonitis, aspiration, hemorrhage, and tube migration. Contraindications include uncorrectable bleeding diatheses, lack of a safe access window into the stomach, massive ascites, anterior gastric wall neoplasm, and the presence of a ventriculoperitoneal shunt.

Notes

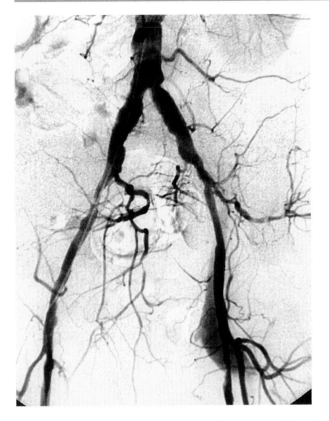 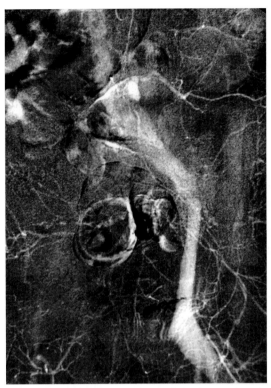

1. What abnormality is depicted in the images above?

2. What are the likely etiologies of such a lesion in this location?

3. What clinical problems can be associated with such a lesion?

4. What is the standard treatment for this lesion?

Femoral Arteriovenous Fistula

1. Early filling of the left iliofemoral venous system during the early arterial phase of the angiogram, indicating a left femoral arteriovenous fistula (AVF).

2. Iatrogenic catheterization injury, trauma, postsurgical complication.

3. Vascular steal of blood from the ipsilateral limb, high-output cardiac failure.

4. Surgical repair of the femoral artery.

References

Perings SM, Kelm M, Jax T. A prospective study on incidence and risk factors of arteriovenous fistulae following transfemoral cardiac catheterization. *Int J Cardiol.* 2003;88:223-228.

Cross-Reference

Vascular and Interventional Radiology: THE REQUISITES, pp 48-52.

Comment

The proper evaluation of an angiogram starts with several important observations: (1) The type of examination should be stated; (2) The catheter position and vascular approach should be noted, and the reader should specify whether nonselective or selective catheter placement has been performed; (3) The reader should be sure to observe whether the image viewed was obtained in the early arterial, late arterial, parenchymal, or venous phases of the dynamic angiographic run.

Complications of arteriography include groin infection, groin hematomas, contrast-related renal dysfunction or allergy, and arterial injuries. Injury to the femoral artery at the puncture site can result in formation of a pseudoaneurysm (which occurs in 1% of angiograms) with or without an arteriovenous fistula. The optimal site of femoral artery puncture is at the femoral head level; at this level, the common femoral artery and vein lie side by side. However, abnormally low punctures of the femoral artery can result in traversal of the femoral vein, with formation of an AVF upon removal of the catheter.

AVFs are usually asymptomatic, but they occasionally enlarge and cause arterial steal or high-output cardiac failure. Surgical ligation of femoral AVFs may be performed in patients who have symptomatic AVFs that fail to spontaneously close.

Notes

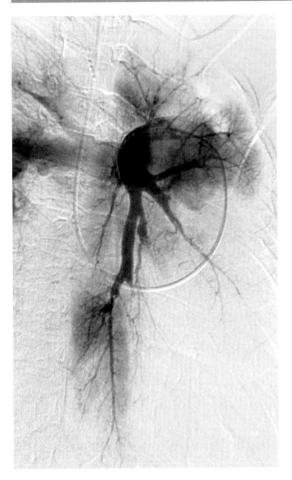
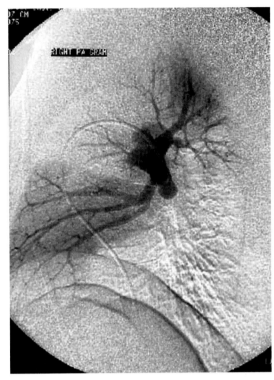

1. Is this more likely an acute or chronic process?

2. What is the most likely cause?

3. Would you expect the pulmonary artery pressures to be normal?

4. How does primary pulmonary hypertension differ on arteriography?

Chronic Pulmonary Embolism

1. Chronic.

2. Thromboembolic disease.

3. No.

4. In primary pulmonary hypertension, acute or organized thrombus is not seen, and there is widespread tortuosity and severe tapering of the distal arterial branches.

Reference

Hansell DM. Small-vessel diseases of the lung: CT–pathologic correlates. *Radiology*. 2002;225:639-653.

Cross-Reference

Vascular and Interventional Radiology: THE REQUISITES, pp 207-208.

Comment

In most patients with acute pulmonary embolism, the emboli resolve partially or completely within several weeks of the event. However, in some patients the emboli do not resolve, and 0.1% to 0.2% of patients develop pulmonary hypertension as a result of multiple episodes of pulmonary embolism. These patients typically present with dyspnea and fatigue that is often progressive. Many patients have no history of deep venous thrombosis or prior known pulmonary embolism.

Angiography remains the gold standard for diagnosis. The findings are characteristic and include enlarged central pulmonary arteries, intra-luminal webs, pulmonary arterial branch stenoses, luminal irregularities, outpouchings often with a rounded-off appearance (as in this case), regional perfusion defects, and frank obstruction of vessels. The mean pulmonary artery pressure is typically elevated.

Notes

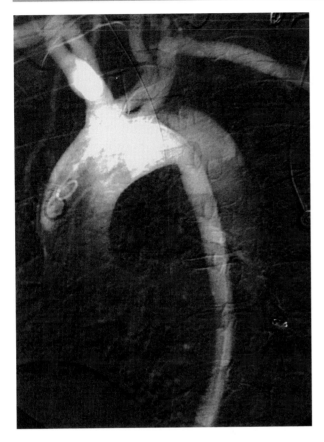 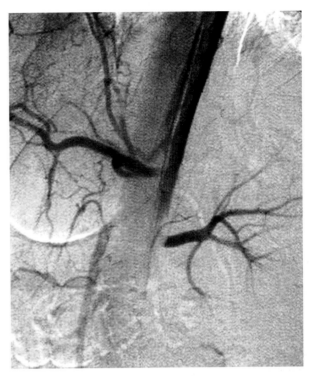

1. What are two commonly used classification systems for this disorder?

2. What imaging modalities are most accurate in the diagnosis of this disorder?

3. Based upon the second image, what complications of this disorder might be expected in this patient?

4. What role does angiography have in the management of this disorder?

Aortic Dissection

1. DeBakey and Stanford.

2. Helical CT, magnetic resonance imaging, and transesophageal echocardiography have superseded angiography in the primary diagnosis of aortic dissection.

3. Renal and/or mesenteric ischemia.

4. Angiography is used primarily to define branch vessel anatomy and lumen of origin in patients undergoing surgery or endovascular therapy.

Reference

Vedantham S, Picus D, Sanchez LA, et al. Percutaneous management of ischemic complications in patients with type-B aortic dissection. *J Vasc Intervent Radiol.* 2003;14:181-193.

Cross-Reference

Vascular and Interventional Radiology: THE REQUISITES, pp 235-239.

Comment

Acute aortic dissection is a life-threatening disease with a mortality of about 1% per hour during the first 48 hours. The definitive diagnosis of aortic dissection is made using helical computed tomography, magnetic resonance imaging, or multiplanar transesophageal echocardiography. Angiography is used when branch vessels must be assessed before surgical aortic repair or endovascular therapy.

Stanford type A dissections involve the ascending aorta with (DeBakey type I) or without (DeBakey type II) concomitant involvement of the descending aorta. Stanford type B dissections (DeBakey type III) involve only the aorta distal to the left subclavian artery. Patients with Stanford type A dissections undergo emergent surgical ascending aortic replacement to prevent the complications of coronary artery occlusion, aortic valvular insufficiency, and rupture into the pericardial sac. Patients with uncomplicated Stanford type B dissections are treated with pharmacologic therapy to reduce the systemic blood pressure and cardiac impulse force.

Treatment options for Stanford type B dissections complicated by branch vessel ischemia include surgical aortic replacement and endovascular therapy. Endovascular interventions include balloon fenestration of the dissection flap, stenting of compromised branch vessels, and placement of aortic stents or stent grafts.

Notes

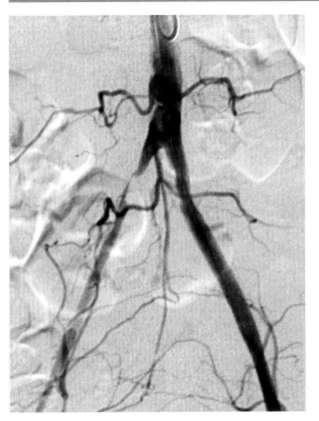 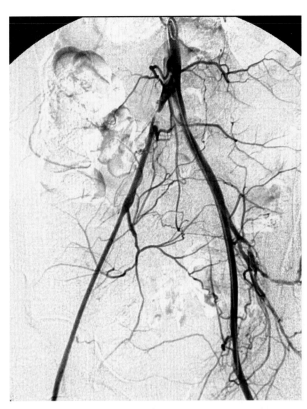

1. How would you describe the findings?

2. What endovascular treatment options might be considered for this lesion?

3. What is the immediate success rate for stenting of this lesion? What is the rate of primary patency at one year? Primary patency at 4 years?

4. What parameters would you use to select an angioplasty balloon and stent?

C A S E 1 9

Iliac Artery Stenosis

1. High-grade stenosis of the proximal right common iliac artery.

2. Percutaneous transluminal angioplasty (PTA) or primary stenting.

3. Technical success rate is 91% to 100%. Primary patency rate is 80% to 90% at 1 year and 75% to 85% at 4 years.

4. An angioplasty balloon should be oversized by approximately 10% of vessel diameter in the iliac arteries. An expanded stent should be 1 to 2 cm longer than the stenotic lesion and 1 mm wider in diameter than normal adjacent vessel lumen.

Reference

Bosch JL, Tetteroo E, Mall WP, et al. Iliac arterial occlusive disease: Cost-effectiveness analysis of stent placement versus percutaneous transluminal angioplasty. *Radiology*. 1998;208:641-648.

Cross-Reference

Vascular and Interventional Radiology: THE REQUISITES, pp 261-270.

Comment

PTA and endoluminal stenting are well-accepted procedures for treating aortoiliac occlusive disease. Treatment is appropriate in patients with claudication that limits lifestyle and in patients with limb-threatening ischemia. Concentric, noncalcified stenoses less than 3 cm long have the best long-term patency after treatment and often respond well to angioplasty alone.

Stent insertion following angioplasty is appropriate for greater than 30% residual stenosis, a residual systolic pressure gradient of greater than 10 mm Hg at rest or greater than 20 mm Hg after administration of a vasodilator, development of a hemodynamically significant dissection, or late restenosis at the angioplasty site. Primary stenting is useful when there is a higher risk of dissection or distal embolization with angioplasty alone—generally for eccentric, calcified plaques or those with small amounts of associated fresh thrombus.

Generally, the secondary patencies of iliac artery angioplasty and stenting are comparable to those of surgical reconstruction but with lower morbidity and mortality rates.

Notes

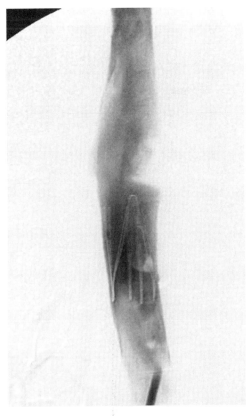

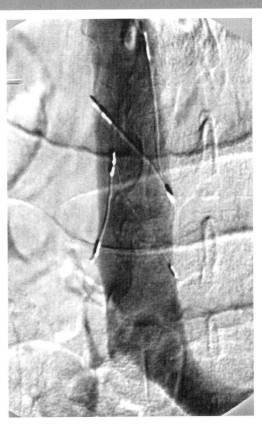

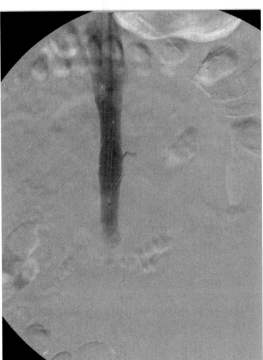

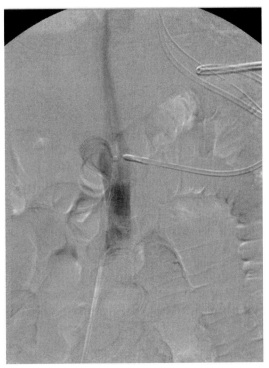

1. Name the devices in the images.

2. Are these devices retrievable?

3. In what situation is it necessary to use the device used in the second image?

4. What are the indications for placement of these devices?

CASE 20

Inferior Vena Cava Filters

1. Vena Tech, bird's nest, TrapEase, and Greenfield inferior vena cava filters.

2. No.

3. Megacava–caval diameter greater than 28 mm.

4. Deep vein thrombosis (DVT) or pulmonary embolism (PE) in patients with contraindications to, complications of, or failure of anticoagulation; patients with poor cardiopulmonary status, for whom a single pulmonary embolus is likely to be fatal; patients with free-floating inferior vena cava (IVC) thrombus.

Reference

Grassi CJ, Swan TL, Cardella JF, et al. Quality improvement guidelines for percutaneous permanent inferior vena cava filter placement for the prevention of pulmonary embolism. *J Vasc Intervent Radiol.* 2001;12: 137-141.

Cross-Reference

Vascular and Interventional Radiology: THE REQUISITES, pp 364-368.

Comment

Different IVC filters vary in terms of their physical characteristics, cost, and deployment method, but all serve to prevent PE in patients with documented lower-extremity DVT and as prophylaxis in selected patients who are at high risk for developing lower-extremity DVT.

An inferior vena cavogram is performed to obtain four specific pieces of information that guide filter selection and placement: (1) Presence of IVC thrombus: This can interfere with proper seating of the filter and might mandate placement at a higher level in the IVC; (2) Location of the lowermost renal vein on each side, because the preferred location of IVC filters is immediately below the renal vein entry; (3) Presence of caval or renal vein anomalies; (4) IVC diameter: Any filter (Greenfield, Boston Scientific; Venatech, Braun; or Simon-Nitinol, Bard) can be inserted into an IVC that measures 18 to 28 mm. However, between 1% and 3% of patients have a megacava, in which the IVC diameter is greater than 28 mm. The TrapEase filter (Cordis) can be inserted into an IVC measuring 18 to 30 mm, and the bird's nest filter (Cook) can be inserted into an IVC measuring up to 40 mm. In the rare situation where the IVC diameter is greater than 40 mm, two filters can be inserted, one into each common iliac vein.

Notes

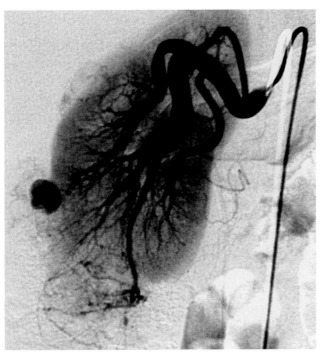

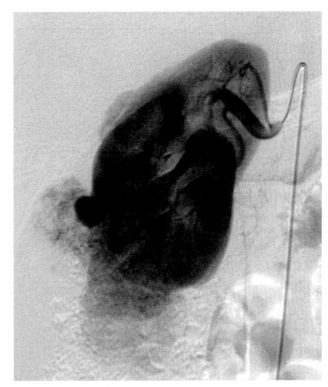

Courtesy of Dr. Daniel Brown.

Courtesy of Dr. Daniel Brown.

1. How would you describe the findings?

2. What is the likely diagnosis?

3. What complication commonly results from these lesions?

4. What congenital syndrome is found with high frequency in patients with these lesions?

C A S E 2 1

Renal Angiomyolipoma

1. Rounded enhancing parenchymal mass lesion.

2. Renal angiomyolipoma (AML).

3. Spontaneous hemorrhage.

4. Tuberous sclerosis is present in 30% to 40% of patients with angiomyolipoma.

Reference

Siegel C. Renal angiomyolipoma: Relationships between tumor size, aneurysm formation, and rupture. *J Urol.* 2003;169:1598-1599.

Cross-Reference

Vascular and Interventional Radiology: THE REQUI-SITES, pp 338-342.

Comment

AMLs are hamartomatous lesions containing fat, smooth muscle, and blood vessels. Approximately 80% of patients with tuberous sclerosis have AMLs, which are often multiple and bilateral in these patients.

AMLs are often diagnosed on cross-sectional imaging owing to the presence of fat within a renal lesion, which nearly always indicates AML. AMLs are usually hypervascular, and this property gives them a characteristic appearance on angiography as well as strong contrast enhancement on MRI and CT. Angiographic features include hypervascularity with large, tortuous feeding arteries arranged circumferentially, occasional small arterial aneurysms, and a sunburst appearance in the parenchymal phase. Arteriovenous shunting does not commonly occur in these lesions. Angiographic differentiation from renal cell carcinoma is usually not definitive.

AMLs are generally treated if they are large or symptomatic or if they bleed spontaneously. Treatment may include surgical resection or percutaneous embolization.

Notes

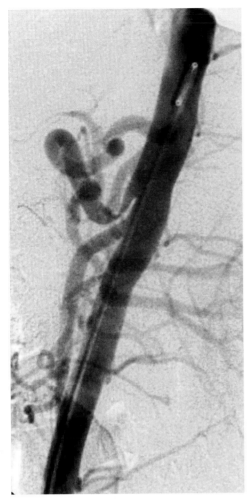

Courtesy of Dr. Sailendra Naidu.

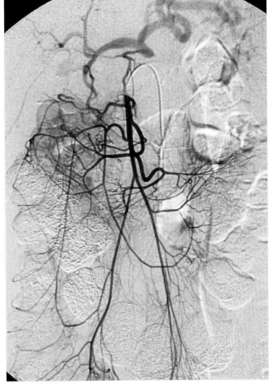

Courtesy of Dr. Sailendra Naidu.

1. What is the diagnosis?

2. What vessel is being selectively injected in the second image? What additional vascular distribution is being filled?

3. Does the obstruction typically worsen during inspiration or expiration?

4. What is the treatment of choice?

Median Arcuate Ligament Syndrome

1. Median arcuate ligament syndrome or celiac artery compression syndrome.

2. Superior mesenteric artery. Celiac artery territory.

3. Expiration.

4. Surgery.

Reference

Douard R, Ettore GM, Chevalier JM, et al. Celiac trunk compression by arcuate ligament and living-related liver transplantation: A two-step strategy for flow-induced enlargement of donor hepatic artery. *Surg Radiol Anat.* 2002;24:327-331.

Cross-Reference

Vascular and Interventional Radiology: THE REQUI-SITES, pp 296-298.

Comment

Median arcuate ligament syndrome or celiac artery compression syndrome is the most common visceral arterial compression syndrome. Patients with this syndrome have extrinsic compression of the celiac artery by the median crus of the diaphragm and/or the celiac neural plexuses and connective tissues. The majority of patients with this diagnosis are young, thin women who are asymptomatic, despite stenoses of more than 50% diameter. However, some patients do develop crampy abdominal pain and malabsorption that has been attributed to celiac artery compression.

The arterial compression usually varies with respiration and worsens with expiration. As in this case, the compression can be severe enough that injection of the superior mesenteric artery produces celiac artery opacification in retrograde fashion via the gastroduodenal and pancreaticoduodenal arteries.

Surgery to enlarge the diaphragmatic hiatus or resect the celiac ganglion is the preferred therapy because this compression does not respond to angioplasty. Stents are contraindicated due to possible device fatigue.

Notes

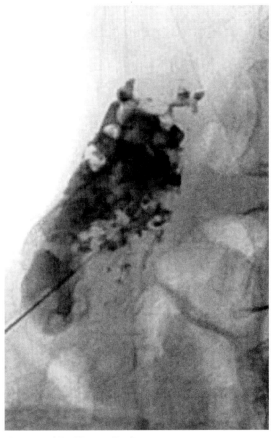

Courtesy of Dr. Thomas Vesely.

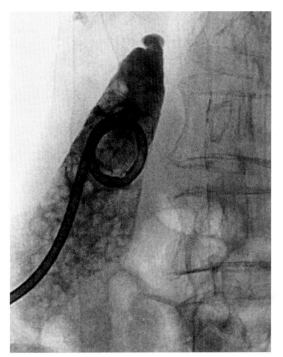

Courtesy of Dr. Thomas Vesely.

1. What are the imaging findings?

2. What treatment was provided?

3. What are the two possible routes of percutaneous drainage?

4. What definitive treatment options exist?

Percutaneous Cholecystostomy

1. Multiple filling defects within the gallbladder and nonfilling of the cystic duct.

2. Percutaneous insertion of a cholecystostomy tube.

3. Transhepatic and through the free peritoneal surface of the gallbladder.

4. Cholecystectomy and percutaneous gallstone removal.

Reference

Menu Y, Vuillerme MP. Non-traumatic abdominal emergencies: Imaging and intervention in acute biliary conditions. *Eur Radiol*. 2002;12:2397-2406.

Cross-Reference

Vascular and Interventional Radiology: THE REQUISITES, pp 589-601.

Comment

The current indications for percutaneous gallbladder drainage include acute calculous or acalculous cholecystitis, access for percutaneous stone dissolution or removal, diagnostic cholangiography, and drainage of the biliary system when the common bile duct is obstructed. For many of these patients the diagnosis of cholecystitis is difficult because the patients are unable to provide history owing to mechanical ventilation or depressed mental status.

There are two different potential routes to percutaneously drain the gallbladder, each with advantages and disadvantages. Transhepatic access is favored by many because there is a reduced incidence of bile leakage into the peritoneum due to the fixation of the gallbladder to the liver surface. However, disadvantages include the potential for liver laceration and bleeding. Therefore, some favor the transperitoneal route. The aspirated bile should be cultured, although negative cultures are found in as many as 40% of patients despite obvious cholecystitis.

To reduce the risk of sepsis, the tube should not be manipulated until the patient improves clinically. Subsequently, cholangiography via the tube is performed to establish cystic and common bile duct patency and to establish the presence or absence of stones that will require further treatment. No drainage catheter should be removed until the underlying problem has resolved and a complete fibrous tract has developed around the catheter from the gallbladder to the skin surface to prevent bile peritonitis.

Notes

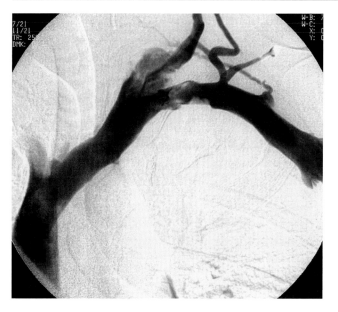 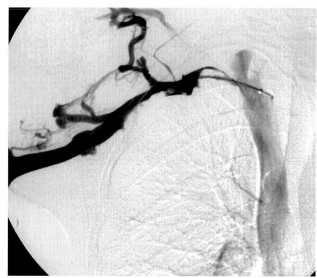

1. Describe the common abnormality seen in these two patients.

2. Name two common etiologies of this lesion.

3. What are the standard treatment options?

4. Is stent placement an effective treatment method?

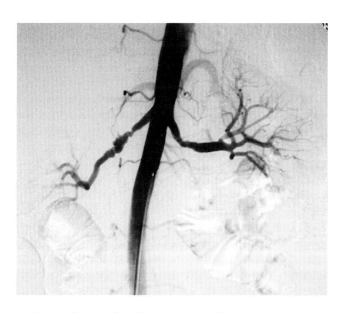 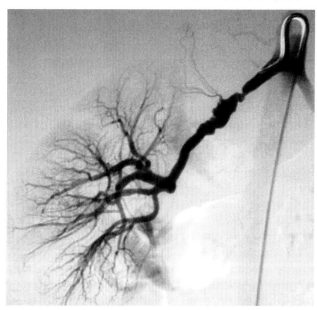

1. How often is this disease bilateral?

2. Is this disease more common in men or in women?

3. What arterial abnormalities can be seen?

4. What is the accepted treatment?

Subclavian Vein Occlusion

1. Subclavian vein stenosis with associated thrombus formation and collateral vein development.

2. Primary subclavian vein occlusion (this case) is caused by thoracic outlet syndrome (Paget-Schroetter syndrome). Secondary subclavian vein occlusion is currently most commonly the result of central venous catheters and pacemakers.

3. Primary subclavian vein occlusion: catheter-directed thrombolysis followed by surgical thoracic outlet decompression and anticoagulation therapy. Secondary subclavian vein occlusion: anticoagulation alone for most patients.

4. No.

Reference
Meissner MH. Axillary–subclavian venous thrombosis. *Rev Cardiovasc Med.* 2002;3(Suppl 2):S76-S83.

Cross-Reference
Vascular and Interventional Radiology: THE REQUISITES, pp 168-173.

Comment
Primary axillosubclavian vein occlusion is caused by mechanical compression of the vein at its point of entry into the thorax. This disorder most commonly is seen in young patients, particularly those with well-developed musculature. The compression induces an intimal reaction in the vein, causing stenosis, which produces symptoms of upper extremity swelling and/or pain. If the occlusion is left undiagnosed, thrombosis often occurs.

The diagnosis of subclavian vein stenosis or thrombosis is usually made by venography. When evaluating a patient for primary axillosubclavian vein occlusion, it is important to perform venographic runs with the arm abducted and during arm abduction with pectoralis flexion. These maneuvers often demonstrate pronounced compression or occlusion of the vein. The disorder is commonly bilateral, so it is important to also evaluate the contralateral upper extremity.

The treatment of primary axillosubclavian occlusion centers on early removal of thrombus via catheter-directed thrombolysis, followed by surgical thoracic outlet decompression. Angioplasty of the underlying subclavian vein stenosis is not performed for fear of further injuring the subclavian vein. Stent placement is contraindicated as initial therapy because of the risk of stent fracture resulting from mechanical compression in this area.

Fibromuscular Dysplasia with Renal Artery Stenosis

1. Two thirds of the time.

2. More common in women than men (ratio 3:1).

3. Alternating areas of stenosis and dilation, focal or long segmental stenoses, aneurysms, dissection.

4. Percutaneous transluminal angioplasty.

Reference
Gowda MS, Loeb AL, Crouse LJ. Complementary roles of color-flow duplex imaging and intravascular ultrasound in the diagnosis of renal artery fibromuscular dysplasia (FMD): Should renal arteriography serve as the "gold standard"? *J Am Coll Cardiol.* 2003;41: 1305-1311.

Cross-Reference
Vascular and Interventional Radiology: THE REQUISITES, pp 327-336.

Comment
FMD is a disorder of unknown cause that most commonly affects the renal arteries. It is the second most common cause of renovascular hypertension (behind atherosclerotic renal artery stenosis). The mid-and distal portions of the main renal artery are most commonly affected, but the entire artery can be involved. Rarely, only the proximal portion is affected. When FMD is unilateral, the right renal artery is more commonly affected. The disease involves renal artery branch vessels in nearly 20%. In less than 5% of cases, only the branch vessels are diseased.

The most common angiographic finding is the string-of-beads appearance seen in the medial fibroplasia variant. Five additional variants have been described. In decreasing order of frequency, these are perimedial fibroplasia, medial hyperplasia, medial dissection, intimal fibroplasia, and adventitial fibroplasia.

In this case, the preferred treatment modality is percutaneous transluminal angioplasty. The expected technical success is similar to angioplasty of atherosclerotic stenoses, but the expected clinical success is better. About 40% of patients are cured of their hypertension, and an additional 40% demonstrate significantly improved blood pressure control following angioplasty. The 5-year patency rates following angioplasty for renal artery FMD are about 90%. Stents are reserved for cases in which iatrogenic dissection occurs following angioplasty.

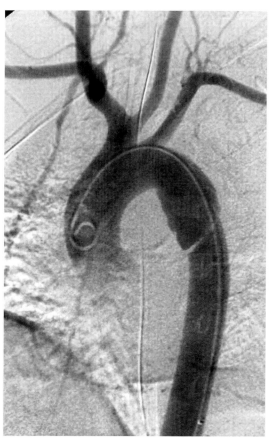

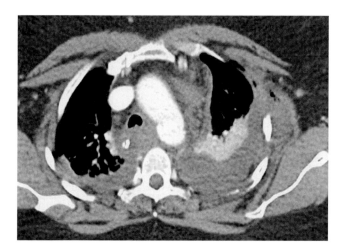

Courtesy of Dr. Daniel Brown.

1. What is the most common angiographic finding in acute traumatic aortic injury (ATAI)?

2. How often is free extravasation seen at angiography?

3. What CT findings may be present in ATAI?

4. How common is great vessel injury with ATAI?

Acute Traumatic Aortic Injury

1. Pseudoaneurysm.

2. Rarely.

3. Mediastinal hematoma, changes in aortic caliber, irregularity of aortic contour, and/or presence of an intimal flap.

4. From 15% to 30% of cases.

Reference

Fattori R, Napoli G, Lovato L, et al. Indications for, timing of, and results of catheter-based treatment of traumatic injury to the aorta. *AJR Am J Roentgenol.* 2002;179:603-609.

Cross-Reference

Vascular and Interventional Radiology: THE REQUI-SITES, pp 239-243.

Comment

ATAI is associated with significant mortality. Aortic rupture is the cause of death in approximately 16% of motor vehicle crashes involving sudden deceleration. Only 15% of patients with ATAI live long enough to survive transfer to the hospital, and the mortality when ATAI is undiagnosed is 30% at 6 hours, 50% at 24 hours, and 90% within 4 months.

Sudden deceleration causes stress at points of maximal fixation in the aorta. The most common traumatic aortic injury seen on angiography (80%) is a laceration just distal to the left subclavian artery at the aortic isthmus, resulting in development of a pseudoaneurysm. The pseudoaneurysm typically appears as a bulge of the aortic contour that can involve the entire circumference of the aorta or only a portion of it. As in the case shown, a linear lucency representing a flap of involved intima and media may be identified. Less-common sites of injury seen on angiography include the ascending aorta (most patients with this injury expire before angiography can be obtained) and the descending thoracic aorta at the diaphragm level.

The treatment of choice for ATAI is emergency surgical aortic repair. In carefully selected patients with associated injuries and comorbidities, stent grafts have also been employed in the management of ATAI.

Notes

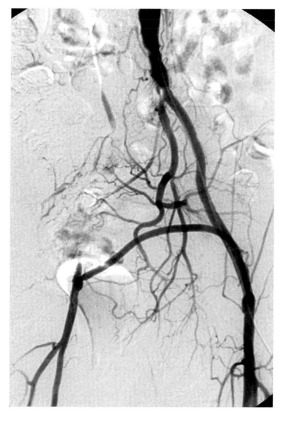
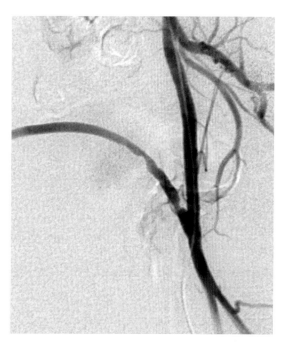

1. What surgical procedure has been performed?

2. What was the probable indication for selecting this procedure?

3. Does this conduit appear normal?

4. What factors are most important in determining long-term patency?

Patent Femorofemoral Bypass Graft

1. Femorofemoral bypass graft.

2. Right common iliac artery occlusion.

3. No. A stenosis is present just beyond the left femoral anastomosis.

4. The severity of disease in the inflow and outflow vessels.

Reference

Nazzal MM, Hoballah JJ, Jacobovicz C, et al. A comparative evaluation of femorofemoral crossover bypass and iliofemoral bypass for unilateral iliac artery occlusive disease. *Angiology*. 1998;49:259-265.

Cross-Reference

Vascular and Interventional Radiology: THE REQUISITES, pp 261-270.

Comment

A femorofemoral bypass graft is an extraanatomic vascular bypass usually used to treat unilateral iliac artery occlusion. Extraanatomic bypass grafts are preferred in patients with unilateral iliac disease, patients who are poor candidates for surgery, patients with severe scarring from prior vascular procedures, patients with current abdominal or groin infections, or patients in whom one limb of an aortobifemoral bypass graft is occluded.

The degree of disease in the native donor and recipient arteries typically determines the long-term patency of the graft. Disease in the donor iliac artery can result in significant flow reduction to both limbs, and in severe cases it can lead to flow reversal in the graft. The presence of superficial femoral artery occlusion reduces the duration of graft patency as well as the likelihood of achieving symptomatic relief. Complications of femorofemoral bypass placement can include graft thrombosis, femoral steal phenomenon, anastomotic pseudoaneurysms, and anastomotic stenoses.

Arteriography is typically performed by catheterizing the donor femoral artery, but other approaches include the axillary artery, the translumbar aorta, and direct graft puncture. Due to the tendency for complications to occur at the anastomoses, it is important to obtain images in different projections to optimally profile these regions.

Notes

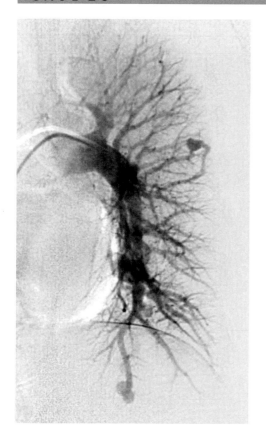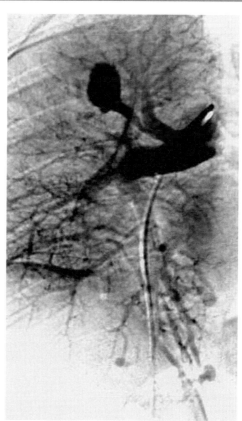

1. What is the most likely diagnosis?

2. What chromosomal abnormality has been identified?

3. How do these patients usually present?

4. What is the embolization material of choice?

Pulmonary Arteriovenous Malformation

1. Hereditary hemorrhagic telangiectasia (HHT), which is also known as Osler–Weber–Rendu syndrome.

2. An abnormality in a gene called *endoglin* on chromosome 9, which codes for an endothelial cell receptor for transforming growth factor β.

3. Stroke, transient ischemic attack, or brain abscess.

4. Coils.

References

Zylak CJ, Eyler WR, Spizamy DL, et al. Developmental lung anomalies in the adult: Radiologic–pathologic correlation. *Radiographics*. 2002;22:S25-S43.

Haitjema T, Disch F, Overtoom TT, et al. Screening family members of patients with hereditary hemorrhagic telangiectasia. *Am J Med*. 1995;99:519-524.

Cross-Reference

Vascular and Interventional Radiology: THE REQUI-SITES, pp 209-212.

Comment

HHT has a reported prevalence of 2 to 3 per 100,000, but it is probably more common because in many patients with mild symptoms it can go undiagnosed. The disorder has a classic triad of mucocutaneous telangiectasias, epistaxis, and autosomal dominant inheritance. About 15% of patients with HHT have pulmonary arteriovenous malformations (AVM), but the risk is higher when there is a family member with a pulmonary AVM.

Although most patients present with the central nervous system manifestations (stroke and brain abscess), the most common clinical manifestations are dyspnea, fatigue, cyanosis, clubbing, and polycythemia.

Treatment options include surgical resection of the involved lung and embolotherapy with coils or detachable balloons. Because the overwhelming majority of pulmonary AVMs have a single feeding artery and a single draining vein, with an intervening thin-walled aneurysm, the goal of therapy is to eliminate arterial inflow. This is in contrast to peripheral (nonpulmonary) AVMs, in which the goal of therapy is to eliminate the nidus when possible. Family members of patients with HHT should undergo screening.

Notes

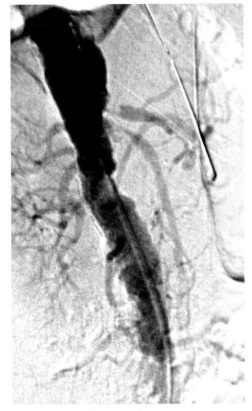

Courtesy of Dr. Thomas Vesely.

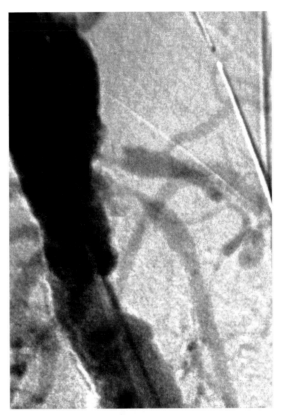

Courtesy of Dr. Thomas Vesely.

1. What abnormality is seen?

2. Is this abnormality likely to be associated with significant symptoms?

3. What specific symptoms are likely to be present?

4. What is the preferred therapy?

Chronic Mesenteric Ischemia

1. Tight origin stenoses of the celiac artery and superior mesenteric artery (SMA).

2. Yes.

3. Intestinal angina (postprandial abdominal pain), food fear, anorexia, weight loss.

4. Surgical aortomesenteric bypass.

References

Park WM, Cherry KJ, Chua HK. Current results of open revascularization for chronic mesenteric ischemia: A standard for comparison. *J Vasc Surg.* 2002;35(5): 853-859.

Matsumoto AH, Angle JF, Spinosa DJ. Percutaneous transluminal angioplasty and stenting in the treatment of chronic mesenteric ischemia: Results and longterm followup. *J Am Coll Surg.* 2002;194(1 Suppl): S22-S31.

Cross-Reference

Vascular and Interventional Radiology: THE REQUISITES, pp 296-298.

Comment

Chronic mesenteric ischemia is less common than acute mesenteric ischemia. The primary cause is atherosclerosis, usually due to aortic plaques that involve the mesenteric artery ostia. These stenoses are typically circumferential and can exhibit post-stenotic dilation. The stenosis can progress to thrombotic occlusion. Most patients are elderly women with risk factors for atherosclerosis. In addition to the classic symptoms listed above, some patients develop nausea, vomiting, and/or diarrhea due to malabsorption. Physical examination is typically unremarkable, although an epigastric bruit may be heard.

It is generally agreed that the diagnosis requires that at least two of the three mesenteric arteries to have significant stenoses or occlusions, as seen in this case, because the splanchnic system has efficient collateral channels. However, milder degrees of stenosis can become symptomatic when cardiac output is reduced. Typically, enlarged collaterals are identified at arteriography because the disease is chronic. The main collaterals between the celiac and SMA circulations are the gastroduodenal and pancreaticoduodenal arteries. The primary collaterals between the SMA and IMA circulations are the marginal artery of Drummond and the arc of Riolan. The IMA can receive flow from the internal iliac arteries via the hemorrhoidal arterial system as well.

Surgical revascularization remains the mainstay of therapy. However, balloon angioplasty with or without stent insertion is an alternative in patients who are poor surgical candidates.

Notes

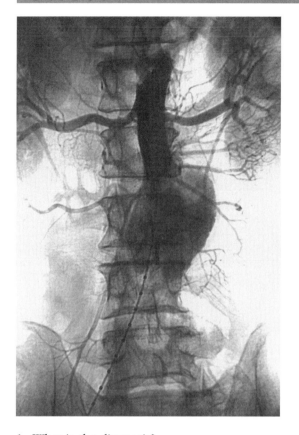

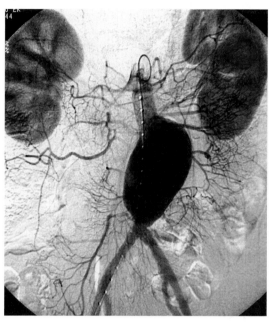

1. What is the diagnosis?

2. What is the best method to diagnose and initially characterize this lesion?

3. For what purpose is angiography being performed?

4. What treatment methods could be used in this patient?

Abdominal Aortic Aneurysm

1. Abdominal aortic aneurysm (AAA).

2. Cross-sectional imaging modalities including ultrasound, computed tomography (CT), and magnetic resonance imaging (MRI).

3. To evaluate the relationship of the aneurysm to branch vessels, to determine if the patient is a candidate for endovascular aneurysm repair, and to make the relevant measurements in the event endovascular repair is used.

4. Surgical repair would likely consist of aortobifemoral bypass graft placement. Endovascular stent-graft placement is another option.

Reference

Golzarian J. Imaging after endovascular repair of abdominal aortic aneurysm. *Abdom Imaging*. 2003;28: 236-243.

Cross-Reference

Vascular and Interventional Radiology: THE REQUISITES, pp 252-261.

Comment

AAAs usually result from atherosclerosis. The most important complications of AAAs are aneurysm rupture and distal embolization. Rupture carries a high mortality rate, and rupture risk increases with larger aneurysm size. AAA treatment is indicated for aneurysms greater than 5 cm in diameter or those that cause distal embolization; a lower size threshold is used in women and in patients with connective tissue disorders.

Imaging diagnosis of AAA is usually made by ultrasonography or CT, both of which are highly sensitive for AAA. These modalities enable precise diameter measurements of the aneurysm and adjacent normal aortic segments to be obtained. In contrast, when thrombus is present within an aneurysm sac, arteriography can be insensitive for the diagnosis of AAA and often underestimates aneurysm diameter. CT angiography is invaluable in obtaining measurements needed for planning stent-graft repair of AAAs. Arteriography is primarily used intraprocedurally to evaluate visceral branch vessel relationships to the aneurysm, to evaluate the suitability of the iliac arteries as access vessels for stent-graft placement, and to enable proper stent-graft device selection and sizing.

The traditional standard treatment of AAA is operative repair with bypass graft placement. In recent years, endovascular stent-graft placement has been employed in patients with suitable anatomy and is clearly indicated in high-risk patients with medical contraindications to aortic surgery. Compared with operative repair, stent grafts have demonstrated diminished periprocedural morbidity and hospital stay.

Notes

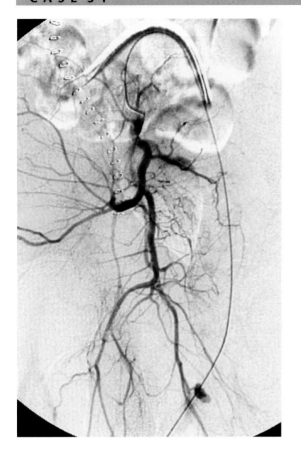

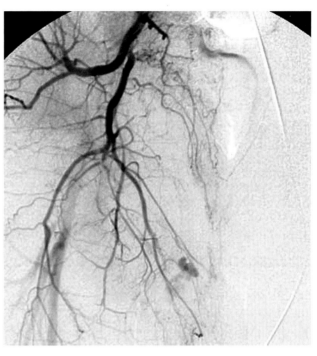

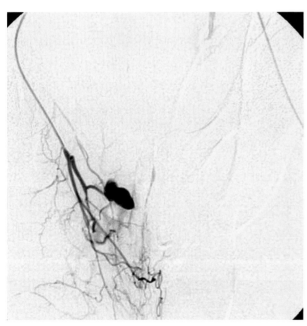

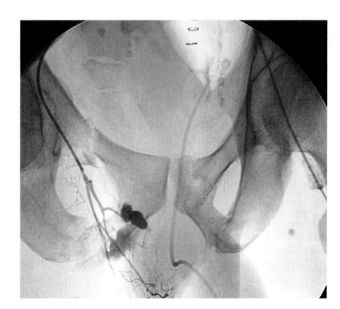

1. What is the arteriographic diagnosis?

2. What additional radiographic findings are present?

3. What is the preferred treatment of the vascular injury?

4. Why is this preferred over surgery?

Pelvic Trauma with Pseudoaneurysm

1. Pseudoaneurysm and active extravasation from a right internal iliac artery branch.

2. Fractures of the right superior and inferior pubic rami and the left pubis.

3. Transcatheter embolization.

4. Operative exploration can lead to uncontrolled bleeding due to loss of the tamponade effect of hematoma below the pelvic peritoneum. Surgery has a high failure rate and an increased risk of infection in this clinical setting.

Reference

Velmahos GC, Toutozas KJ, Vassiliu P, et al. A prospective study on the safety and efficacy of angiographic embolization for pelvic and visceral injuries. *J Trauma*. 2002;53:303-308.

Cross-Reference

Vascular and Interventional Radiology: THE REQUISITES, pp 277-280.

Comment

Blunt pelvic trauma usually results from motor vehicle crashes, falls from a height, and crush injuries. Approximately 10% of patients with pelvic fractures have pelvic bleeding that requires therapy. These patients are often hypotensive and have multiple organ injuries. Prompt treatment of active hemorrhage is necessary because mortality is primarily related to hemorrhage and sepsis. Commonly injured vessels are the superior gluteal and internal pudendal arteries, and injury results from adjacent pelvic fractures.

The focus of extravasation may be evident on nonselective angiography of the abdominal aorta. However, it is necessary to select both internal iliac arteries to exclude a vascular injury, and the entire pelvis including the femoral regions should be studied because there may be multiple sites of bleeding. Arteriographic findings can include contrast extravasation, pseudoaneurysm, vasospasm, vascular occlusion, and hematoma (displacement, compression, and/or stretching of arterial branches), and/or arteriovenous fistula.

Transcatheter embolization with coils or Gelfoam is the preferred treatment. Both internal iliac artery branches should be treated if the bleeding site is midline so as to prevent continued hemorrhage from collateral flow. Selective embolization is preferred if possible, but in the unstable patient, embolization of the proximal internal iliac artery may be necessary and is usually well tolerated.

Notes

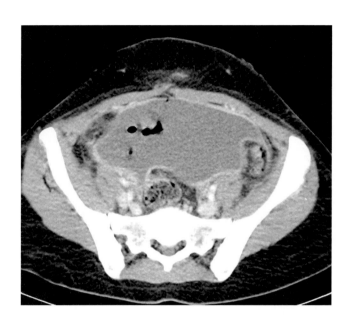 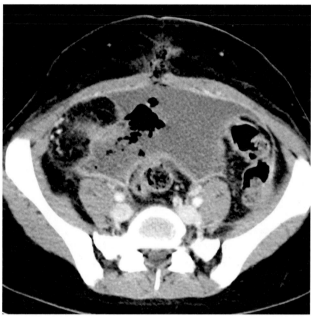

1. What is the most likely diagnosis based on this CT examination performed in a young woman with fevers and leukocytosis 8 days following colorectal surgery?

2. What are the main treatment options?

3. What preprocedure management is appropriate?

4. What criteria determine the timing of catheter removal?

Percutaneous Abscess Drainage

1. Intraabdominal abscess.

2. Percutaneous catheter drainage or surgical exploration and washout.

3. History and physical, evaluation of coagulation profile, and administration of antibiotics appropriate to cover the likely infectious organisms.

4. Clinical improvement of the patient, reduction of drain catheter output, resolution of the fluid collection, collapse of the cavity, and absence of fistula.

Reference

Lee MJ. Non-traumatic abdominal emergencies: Imaging and intervention in sepsis. *Eur Radiol.* 2002;12: 2172-2179.

Cross-Reference

Vascular and Interventional Radiology: THE REQUI-SITES, pp 489-513.

Comment

Percutaneous catheter drainage of an infected fluid collection is a common procedure performed by the interventional radiologist. Percutaneous drainage has nearly replaced surgical drainage as the treatment of choice for abscesses or other fluid collections because it is less invasive and has lower morbidity and expense. A safe route to the fluid collection is required for percutaneous drainage, and typically fluoroscopy, ultrasound, or CT can be used to guide safe passage of the needle so that vital structures are not transgressed. The best candidate fluid collections are those that are unilocular, well-defined, and free-flowing. More-complex collections (e.g., multilocular or debris laden) can be drained percutaneously, but complete drainage may be slow or impossible.

Because drainage of infected collections can cause transient bacteremia, all patients should receive antibiotics before and after the procedure. A sample of the fluid should be acquired for culture, so that the antibiotics can be tailored to treat the organisms involved. The clinical condition of most patients improves significantly within 24 to 48 hours of effective drainage. Follow-up imaging is necessary to establish satisfactory drainage and exclude the presence of undrained components or fistulas, particularly when the clinical condition does not improve or there is continued daily output that does not taper in volume

Notes

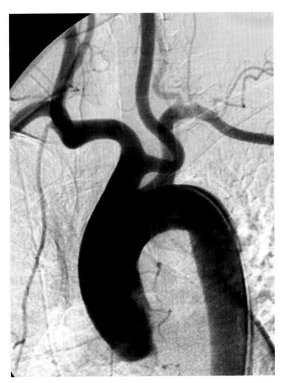

Courtesy of Dr. Daniel Brown.

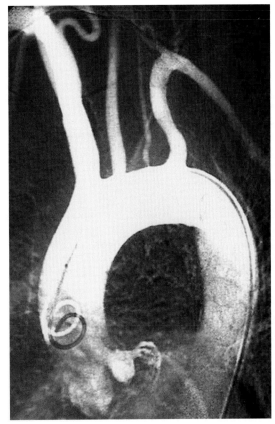

Courtesy of Dr. Daniel Brown.

1. What anatomic variant is depicted in the first image?

2. What caconym is often used to describe this variant?

3. What anatomic variant is depicted in the second image?

4. How common are these two variants?

Variant Anatomy: Aortic Arch

1. Common origin of the brachiocephalic artery and left common carotid artery.

2. Bovine arch.

3. Origin of the left vertebral artery directly from the aortic arch.

4. Bovine arch in 15% to 25% of the population, left vertebral artery origin from the aortic arch in 5% of the population.

Reference

Morgan-Hughes G, Roobottom C, Ring N. Anomalous aortic arch anatomy: Three dimensional visualisation with multislice computed tomography. *Postgrad Med J*. 2003;79(929):167.

Cross-Reference

Vascular and Interventional Radiology: THE REQUI-SITES, pp 219-224.

Comment

Normally there are three branch vessels arising from the aortic arch. In order, these are the brachiocephalic artery, the left common carotid artery, and the left subclavian artery. Although this is the typical configuration, it is seen in only about 70% of patients. Multiple anatomic variants comprise the remainder. The most common of these is a common origin of the right brachiocephalic and left common carotid arteries. Following this in decreasing order of frequency include direct origin of the left vertebral artery from the aortic arch, common origin of the common carotid arteries, presence of two brachiocephalic arteries, and separate origin of each of the four great vessels from the aortic arch.

Notes

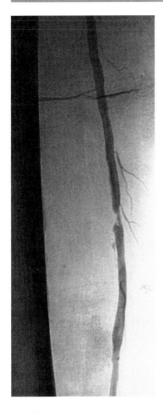 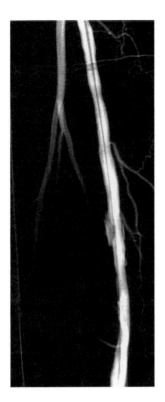

1. What procedure was performed between the times at which the two images above were obtained?

2. Based upon the first image alone, if no other vascular lesions were present, what symptom did the patient likely have?

3. Based upon the first image alone, if no other vascular lesions were present, what was the patient's ankle-brachial index (ABI) likely to be?

4. Is the procedure that was performed associated with a higher patency rate than the surgical procedure that would be used to treat this problem?

Superficial Femoral Artery Stenosis

1. Percutaneous balloon angioplasty of a right superficial femoral artery stenosis.

2. Right calf claudication.

3. Likely 0.5 to 0.9.

4. No. In the superficial femoral artery, the expected patency following angioplasty is lower than that associated with femoropopliteal bypass. However, the morbidity of angioplasty compares favorably with that of surgery.

Reference

Hunink M, Wong J, Donaldson M, et al. Revascularization for femoropopliteal disease: A decision and cost-effectiveness analysis. *JAMA*. 1995;274:167-171.

Cross-Reference

Vascular and Interventional Radiology: THE REQUISITES, pp 419-428.

Comment

In general, patients with a single vascular level of disease are likely to experience intermittent claudication without rest pain and are likely to have an ABI of 0.5 to 0.9. Patients with rest pain nearly always have more than one level of vascular disease (for example, iliac artery disease and femoral artery disease), and they typically have an ABI under 0.4.

The major indications for invasive treatment of lower-extremity atherosclerotic disease are limb-threatening rest pain, lifestyle-limiting intermittent claudication, and the presence of a lesion that is suspected of being a source of distal embolization.

The expected 5-year patency of a femoropopliteal bypass graft is 50% to 80% depending upon the level of the distal anastomosis and the quality of the runoff vessels. In contrast, the expected 2-year patency of a superficial femoral artery angioplasty procedure is 50% to 70%, with 5-year patency well under 50%. However, the morbidity of angioplasty is significantly lower than that of surgical bypass grafting, and bypass can always be performed following failure of angioplasty or recurrence after it. For these reasons, patients with isolated superficial femoral artery stenoses thought to be amenable to angioplasty (short, concentric stenoses) are often treated with angioplasty first. Nitinol stents can be used to improve patency in patients who have poor technical results with angioplasty or in more-complex lesions.

Notes

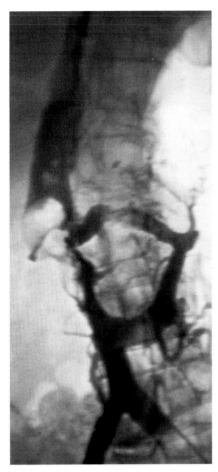

Courtesy of Dr. Thomas Vesely.

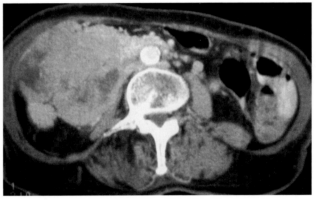

Courtesy of Dr. Thomas Vesely.

1. What pathologic abnormality is present?

2. What normal variant is present?

3. If an inferior vena cava (IVC) filter is required, where should it be placed?

4. Is this patient at significant risk for pulmonary embolism?

Inferior Vena Cava Thrombosis

1. Acute thrombosis of the inferior vena cava.

2. Circumaortic left renal vein.

3. Suprarenal IVC.

4. Yes.

Reference

Razavi MK, Hansch EC, Kee ST, et al. Chronically occluded inferior venae cavae: Endovascular treatment. *Radiology*. 2000;214:133-138.

Cross-Reference

Vascular and Interventional Radiology: THE REQUISITES, pp 361-364.

Comment

The etiologies of IVC thrombosis include IVC filter placement, abdominal malignancy with mass effect upon the IVC, sepsis, dehydration, and hypercoagulability. Depending upon collateral formation and the extent of venous involvement, the symptoms can include bilateral lower-extremity and lower-body wall edema and lower-extremity pain. Anticoagulation therapy is typically given to minimize the acute symptomatology and to decrease the substantial risk of pulmonary embolism. In carefully selected patients, catheter-directed thrombolysis can be used to achieve venous recanalization as well.

Abdominal tumors can cause IVC thrombosis via compression or outright invasion. The most common histology of such lesions is renal cell carcinoma, although other lesions such as hepatocellular carcinoma, adrenal carcinoma, nodal metastases, and IVC leiomyomas (as in this case) can cause IVC thrombosis as well. In patients with renal cell carcinoma, the presence of IVC involvement does not usually preclude surgical resection.

Notes

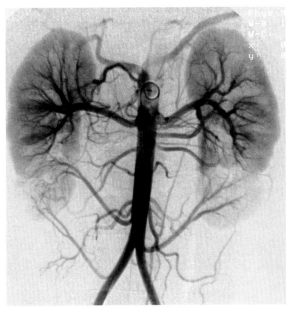

Courtesy of Dr. Thomas Vesely.

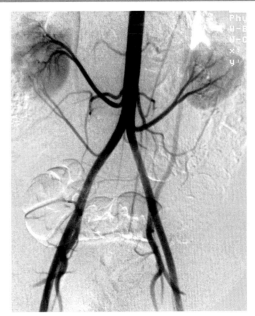

Courtesy of Dr. Thomas Vesely.

1. Why might the study above have been performed?

2. What main findings are present?

3. How often does this anatomic variant occur?

4. With conventional anatomy, which kidney is harvested for transplant and why?

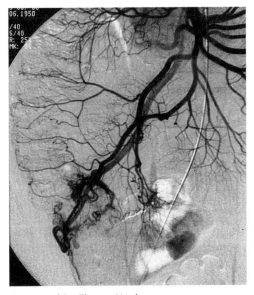

Courtesy of Dr. Thomas Vesely.

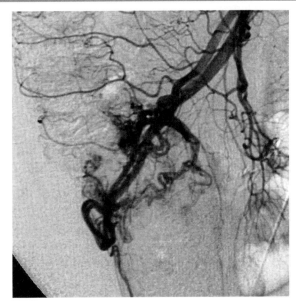

Courtesy of Dr. Thomas Vesely.

1. What is the diagnosis?

2. Where is this abnormality typically located?

3. How common is this abnormality?

4. What percentage of lower gastrointestinal (GI) bleeds are attributable to this diagnosis?

CASE 36

Variant Anatomy: Multiple Renal Arteries

1. Transplant donor, evaluation for possible renal artery stenosis (due to hypertension or chronic renal insufficiency).

2. Three renal arteries on the right and two renal arteries on the left.

3. About 30% of patients have more than one renal artery.

4. All other factors being equal, the left kidney is generally harvested for transplantation because the longer left renal vein facilitates easier anastomosis.

Reference

Liem YS, Kock MC, Ijzermans JN, et al. Living renal donors: Optimizing the imaging strategy–decision and cost-effectiveness analysis. *Radiology*. 2003;226:53-62.

Cross-Reference

Vascular and Interventional Radiology: THE REQUI-SITES, pp 323-325.

Comment

Patients being considered as donors for renal transplantation generally undergo preoperative angiographic evaluation directed at determining several specific pieces of information. (1) The size and number of renal arteries on each side and the presence of any anatomic variants: Generally, kidneys with a single renal artery of significant size are preferred; (2) The presence of early bifurcation of the renal artery: This is important because there must be sufficient room to place a clamp (which measures approximately 1 cm in width) across the donor main renal artery before its division; (3) The presence of stenosis or any evidence of fibromuscular dysplasia: Patients with these disorders are not considered candidates for transplantation; (4) The presence of parenchymal or ureteral anomalies that are not detected on other imaging examinations.

Multiple renal arteries occur in 30% of patients, and they represent the most common anomaly of the renal arteries. Accessory renal arteries most commonly arise from the aorta inferior to the main renal artery, but they can arise anywhere in the abdominal aorta or from the iliac arteries, as in the case depicted above. If the flush aortogram does not clearly demonstrate what parenchymal distribution is supplied by a particular artery suspected of providing renal supply, then selective arteriography can be performed to clarify this.

In recent years, many institutions rely instead upon noninvasive modalities such as MR angiography or CT arteriography to evaluate renal donors.

CASE 37

Angiodysplasia

1. Angiodysplasia.

2. Right colon, especially the cecum.

3. About 2% of autopsies.

4. From 3% to 5%.

Reference

Junquera F, Quiroga S, Saperas E, et al. Accuracy of helical computed tomographic angiography for the diagnosis of colonic angiodysplasia. *Gastroenterology*. 2000;119:293-299.

Cross-Reference

Vascular and Interventional Radiology: THE REQUI-SITES, pp 298-304.

Comment

Angiodysplasia is a vascular abnormality that may be the cause of chronic intermittent GI bleeding or, rarely, acute massive bleeding in up to 50% of persons older than 55 years. However, because it has been identified incidentally in 15% of nonbleeding patients at mesenteric angiography, the presence of angiodysplasia does not confirm that it is the source of bleeding. Active contrast extravasation is only identified in 10% of cases. Therefore, in the evaluation of GI bleeding, one should diligently search for an alternate cause of bleeding if angiodysplasia without active extravasation is identified.

Although these lesions can be located anywhere along the GI tract, they are typically located within the right colon and particularly within the cecum. They range in size from very tiny to very large, as in this case. The imaging characteristics include a vascular tuft or tangle of vessels with early, intense filling of the draining vein that then slowly empties. To make the diagnosis one needs to see simultaneous opacification of the artery and vein that, because they run in parallel, typically creates a tram-track appearance. This lesion can be missed at colonoscopy, so angiography is very useful in diagnosis.

Because of the abnormal vessels, bleeding from angiodysplasia is typically not responsive to vasopressin infusion. Surgical resection is curative. Embolization has been attempted with variable success.

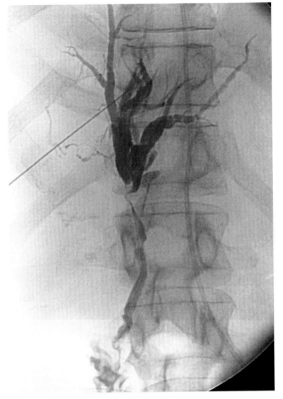

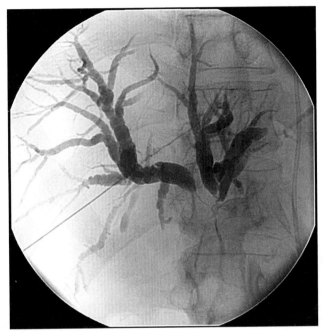

Courtesy of Dr. Daniel Brown.   *Courtesy of Dr. Daniel Brown.*

1. What examination is depicted?

2. Where should the needle be inserted to evaluate the right hepatic ducts?

3. What is the differential diagnosis?

4. What are the major complications of this procedure?

Cholangiocarcinoma (Klatskin Tumor)

1. Percutaneous transhepatic cholangiogram (PTC).

2. Low intercostal approach (preferably below the 10th rib) in the right midaxillary line.

3. Cholangiocarcinoma, gallbladder cancer, hepatocellular carcinoma, metastases, extrinsic adenopathy.

4. Biliary sepsis and hemorrhage.

Reference

Szklaruk J, Tamm E, Charnsangevej C. Preoperative imaging of biliary tract cancers. *Surg Oncol Clin N Am*. 2002;11:865-876.

Cross-Reference

Vascular and Interventional Radiology: THE REQUISITES, pp 558-579.

Comment

PTC has largely been replaced by endoscopic retrograde cholangiopancreatography (ERCP). The primary indications for PTC are evaluation and treatment of biliary obstructive disease in symptomatic patients who are not amenable to or who fail ERCP.

Bacterial overgrowth is common in patients with biliary obstruction. Therefore, all patients should receive preprocedure antibiotics to cover gram-negative species, even in the absence of overt signs and symptoms of cholangitis. A bile duct sample should be sent for culture. Aspirated bile can be sent for cytologic analysis when neoplasm is suspected. Material can also be acquired using a brush biopsy device or fine needle aspiration. Larger specimens can be obtained using biopsy forceps or atherectomy devices.

If it is necessary to drain the liver percutaneously, a peripheral biliary radical should be selected from the cholangiogram images for needle and subsequent catheter insertion, if the initial needle entry site is unfavorable. Manipulation should be minimized in patients with signs and symptoms of suppurative cholangitis, and in these patients temporary external drainage is preferred. Definitive internal drainage via internal–external biliary drains or internal stents may be delayed several days to allow resolution of cholangitis.

Contraindications to PTC include uncorrectable coagulopathy and massive ascites.

Notes

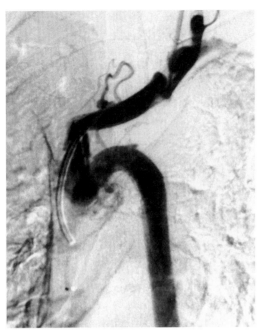

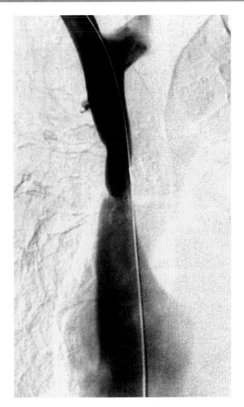

Courtesy of Dr. Thomas Vesely.

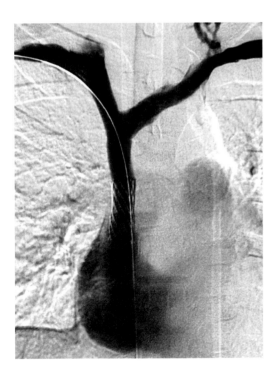

1. What symptoms are experienced by the patient with the venograms in the first two images?

2. What is the most common underlying etiology of this syndrome?

3. What other risk factors can contribute to the development of this abnormality?

4. What endovascular treatment modality is effective in treating this abnormality?

Superior Vena Cava Obstruction

1. Swelling of the face, head, neck, and arms.

2. Intrathoracic malignancy.

3. Central venous catheters, pacemakers, prior radiation therapy.

4. Placement of an endovascular stent (seen in the third image).

References

Nicholson AA, Ettles DF, Arnold A, et al. Treatment of malignant superior vena cava obstruction: Metal stents or radiation therapy. *J Vasc Intervent Radiol.* 1997;8:781-788.

Vedantham S. Endovascular strategies for superior vena cava obstruction. *Tech Vasc Intervent Radiol.* 2000;3:29-39.

Cross-Reference

Vascular and Interventional Radiology: THE REQUI-SITES, pp 173-174.

Comment

Patients with superior vena cava obstruction (SVCO) commonly experience pronounced facial and arm swelling, headaches, hoarseness, dysphagia, and dyspnea. In severe cases, SVCO can cause syncope, visual and cognitive disturbances, seizures, and even coma. The most common cause of SVCO is intrathoracic malignancy, commonly bronchogenic carcinoma or lymphoma. Other risk factors for the development of SVCO include the use of central venous catheters, pacemakers, and prior radiation therapy.

Patients with malignant SVCO are typically treated with external-beam irradiation with or without adjunctive chemotherapy depending upon tumor histology and stage. This approach produces symptomatic improvement in 60% to 75% of patients within 2 to 4 weeks. Patients with benign causes of SVCO are usually treated with anticoagulation, and selected patients are offered surgical venous bypass.

Endovascular methods have been used to treat SVCO with good short-term success. When SVCO is caused by SVC stenosis without thrombus formation (as in the top right-hand image), endovascular stents can be placed (bottom image). When SVC thrombosis is present, catheter-directed thrombolysis can first be used to remove the thrombus before the stent is placed. Response to endovascular therapy occurs in 95% of patients within a few days.

Notes

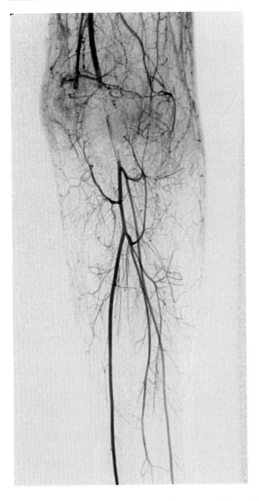
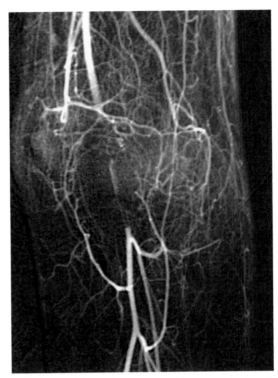

1. What are the hard clinical signs of a major arterial injury?

2. Is the presence of a peripheral pulse a reliable indicator that arterial injury is not present?

3. Should the abnormality in the images be treated percutaneously?

4. What angiographic findings of traumatic arterial injury are commonly seen?

Traumatic Brachial Artery Occlusion

1. Pulsatile bleeding, expanding hematoma, pulse deficits, distal ischemia, bruit or thrill at the injury site.

2. No.

3. No. Surgical thrombectomy with brachial artery repair is indicated.

4. Intimal defects indicating dissection, intraluminal filling defects indicating thrombosis, vasospasm, extrinsic mass effect or defects suggesting extrinsic or intramural hematoma, pseudoaneurysm, distal embolization of thrombus, frank contrast extravasation indicating major active bleeding or arterial transection, and early venous filling indicative of arteriovenous fistula formation.

Reference

Soto JA, Munera F, Morales C. Focal arterial injuries of the proximal extremities: Helical CT arteriography as the initial method of diagnosis. *Radiology*. 2001;218:188-194.

Cross-Reference

Vascular and Interventional Radiology: THE REQUISITES, pp 158-159.

Comment

When hard clinical signs of upper extremity arterial injury are present, angiography should be performed promptly to guide surgical repair. When hard clinical signs are absent, indications for angiography include a shotgun blast etiology, a bullet following the course of a major artery over a long segment, history of peripheral vascular disease in the involved limb, thoracic outlet injury location, or the presence of extensive injury to bone or soft tissue. Angiography can be performed electively in proximity injuries.

Catheter angiography is the gold standard for evaluating injuries to upper-extremity arteries. Guidewire and catheter manipulation within the area suspected of being injured should be avoided whenever possible in order to avoid inducing vasospasm that could be mistaken for an injury. Angiography provides information about the presence and location of arterial injury as well as the extent of injury. The presence of unsuspected injuries and the etiology of any pulse deficits might also be indicated by angiography.

Common pitfalls in diagnosis include mistaking lacerated intima for thrombus or embolus, mistaking vasospasm for occlusion, and missing an intimal injury owing to dense contrast or overlying bone. Two projections should be used for a complete study.

Notes

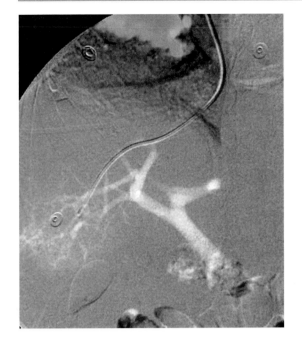

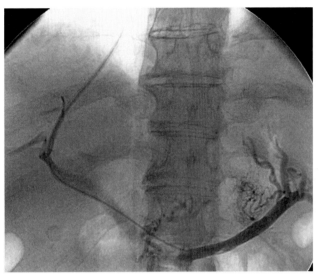

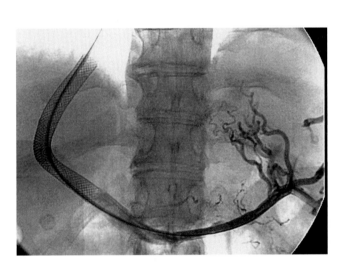

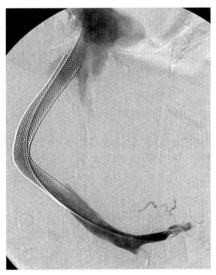

1. What are the primary indications for the procedure depicted above?

2. How was the first image above obtained?

3. What portosystemic gradient is associated with an increased risk for gastroesophageal variceal hemorrhage?

4. What adjunctive procedures are commonly performed during this procedure?

CASE 41

Transjugular Intrahepatic Portosystemic Shunt

1. Intractable ascites, bleeding gastroesophageal varices that have failed endoscopic management, and refractory hepatic hydrothorax.

2. Carbon dioxide portography performed by injection through a catheter in the right hepatic vein.

3. Greater than 12 mm Hg.

4. Percutaneous drainage of ascites and/or coil embolization of persistent varices.

References

Boyer TD. Transjugular intrahepatic portosystemic shunt: Current status. *Gastroenterology.* 2003;124: 1700-1710.

Biecker E, Roth F, Heller J, et al. Prognostic role of the initial portal pressure gradient reduction after TIPS in patients with cirrhosis. *Eur J Gastroenterol Hepatol.* 2007;19:846-852.

Cross-Reference

Vascular and Interventional Radiology: THE REQUISITES, pp 391-399.

Comment

A transjugular intrahepatic portosystemic shunt (TIPS) is intended to decrease portal vein pressures in patients with portal hypertension by creating a conduit for blood to bypass the hepatic parenchyma and enter the systemic circulation. Therefore, the best candidates for TIPS are those who either have recurrent ascites requiring repeated large-volume paracentesis or bleeding gastroesophageal varices that have failed initial endoscopic treatment or have recurred despite treatment.

A long curved needle is passed through the hepatic parenchyma from a hepatic vein (usually the right hepatic vein) to a nearby portal vein (usually the right portal vein). When portal vein access is successfully attained, pressures are measured in the portal vein and right atrium, the hepatic tract is dilated, and a stent graft is inserted. Post-TIPS portal vein and right atrial pressures are then acquired. The goal of TIPS placement is to reduce this portosystemic gradient to less than 12 mm Hg to decrease the risk of gastroesophageal variceal hemorrhage. The portosystemic gradient should be reduced to between 6 and 8 mm Hg if the indication is intractable ascites.

The decision to place a TIPS is best made in conjunction with the hepatologist, gastroenterologist, and transplant surgeon, because not all patients benefit from a TIPS, and some patients worsen after TIPS placement. The Childs-Pugh classification system and the MELD scoring system are used to classify patients and gain an estimate of the relative benefits and risks of the procedure.

Notes

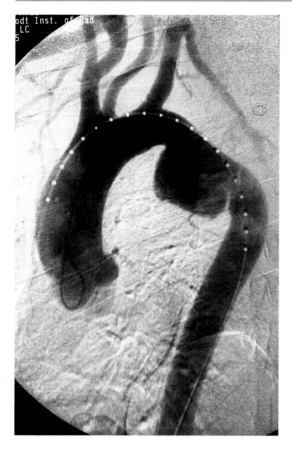

1. What is the diagnosis?

2. What is the likely etiology of this particular lesion?

3. What is the purpose of the radiopaque markers on the catheter?

4. Can this lesion be treated in an endovascular fashion?

Thoracic Aortic Aneurysm

1. Thoracic aortic aneurysm.

2. Atherosclerosis or prior trauma.

3. The marker catheter is used to provide precise longitudinal measurements of the length of the aneurysm and its proximal and distal necks.

4. Yes, using a stent graft.

Reference
Mitchell RS. Stent grafts for the thoracic aorta: A new paradigm? *Ann Thorac Surg.* 2002;74(5):S1818-S1820.

Cross-Reference
Vascular and Interventional Radiology: THE REQUISITES, pp 228-235.

Comment
Thoracic aortic aneurysms (TAAs) are commonly the result of atherosclerotic disease, although they can also result from trauma, connective tissue disorders, syphilis, infection, and other conditions. The main complication of TAAs is that of rupture, which occurs in 30% of aneurysms greater than 6 cm in diameter. For these reasons, TAAs 5.5 to 6.0 cm in diameter are generally repaired surgically. In female patients and those with connective tissue disorders, TAAs tend to rupture at smaller diameters, and these patients are therefore usually referred earlier for surgical repair.

The diagnosis of TAA is generally made using CT or MRI. Angiography is rarely used for the diagnosis of TAA, and it does not provide accurate aneurysm diameter measurements in comparison with CT and MRI. However, angiography provides fairly accurate measurements of the length of the aorta and the degree of angulation in the proximal neck of the aneurysm, and it accurately depicts the aneurysm's relationship to the origins of the great vessels. These findings can be extremely important in surgical planning and in selecting a device and access route for endovascular stent-graft repair.

The most important drawbacks of surgical TAA repair are significant rates of perioperative mortality (6%–12%), paraplegia (3%–16%), and cardiopulmonary complications (5%–30%). Early results suggest that significant improvements in perioperative mortality and morbidity are likely to be achieved with endovascular repair, although the durability of these procedures is not known.

Notes

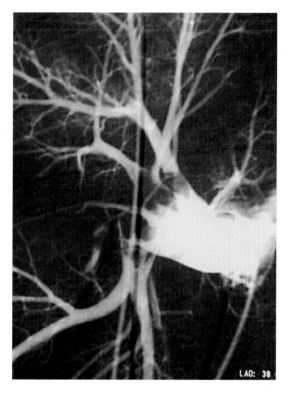

1. What is the diagnosis?

2. What is the most common and reliable angiographic finding in this disorder?

3. What electrocardiographic finding is of particular concern in a patient who is about to undergo pulmonary arteriography, and how is this problem circumvented?

4. What are normal right atrium, right ventricle, and pulmonary artery pressures?

Acute Pulmonary Embolism

1. Acute pulmonary embolism.

2. Intraluminal filling defect at least partially surrounded by contrast material.

3. Left bundle branch block. A transvenous pacer can be placed.

4. Right atrium: 0–8 mm Hg mean. Right ventricle: 15–30 mm Hg systolic, 0–8 mm Hg diastolic. Pulmonary artery: 15–30 mm Hg systolic, 3–12 mm Hg diastolic.

Reference

Harvey RB, Gester WB, Hrung JM, et al. Accuracy of CT angiography versus pulmonary angiography in the diagnosis of acute pulmonary embolism: Evaluation of the literature with summary ROC curve analysis. *Acad Radiol.* 2000;7:786-797.

Cross-Reference

Vascular and Interventional Radiology: THE REQUI-SITES, pp 202-207.

Comment

With the advent of spiral CT angiography, pulmonary arteriography is being performed much less often in the diagnosis of pulmonary embolism. Pulmonary arteriography has a negative predictive value of nearly 100% for vascular thromboembolism within 3 months.

The range of angiographic findings in acute pulmonary embolism includes abrupt vessel cutoff, intraluminal filling defects manifested by the tram-track sign, wedge-shaped parenchymal oligemia, absence of a draining vein from the affected segment, arterial collaterals, and hypervascularity of an infarcted segment. Pulmonary emboli are typically multiple and bilateral, and they tend to lodge in the lower lobe vessels.

The accuracy of pulmonary arteriography can be optimized with attention to several facts. Emboli lyse rapidly, so arteriography should be performed within 24 to 48 hours of symptoms. Multiple projections of both lungs should be obtained. Ventilation–perfusion scans and CT can be used to focus the examination to suspicious areas. Careful attention to small vessels, particularly in the lower lobes, is critical because many patients only have subsegmental emboli. Emboli can be missed because of overlapping vessels, small size of the emboli, or respiratory or patient motion, so additional imaging, including oblique or magnification views or selective vessel injection, may be necessary. False positives can occur from overlapping of vessels, mock lines, cystic air spaces, or poor opacification.

Notes

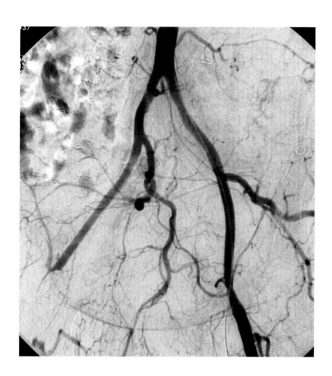
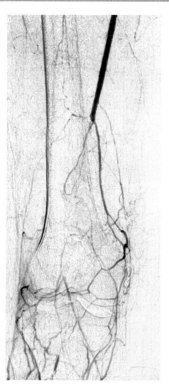

1. What are the most common causes of acute lower-extremity ischemia?

2. What is the diagnosis in this case?

3. What angiographic signs suggest this diagnosis?

4. What is the most common source of arterial emboli?

Embolic Femoral Artery Occlusion

1. Embolization, thrombosis of atherosclerotic native arteries, and occlusion of bypass grafts.

2. Acute emboli to the right common femoral artery and superficial femoral artery.

3. Abrupt vessel cutoff, meniscus configuration of cutoff, lack of significant atherosclerotic disease elsewhere, poor development of collaterals.

4. Embolization of left-heart thrombus.

Reference

Ouriel K. Current status of thrombolysis for peripheral arterial occlusive disease. *Ann Vasc Surg.* 2002;16: 797-804.

Cross-Reference

Vascular and Interventional Radiology: THE REQUI-SITES, pp 429-433.

Comment

Patients with acute limb ischemia typically present with a cold painful leg with pallor, cyanosis, and/or paresthesias. A careful pulse examination often suggests the level of obstruction. Profound sensory loss, muscle weakness, or paralysis are concerning for irreversible ischemia. Most macroemboli lodge near branch points in the femoral or popliteal arteries.

The role of angiography in the evaluation of acute limb ischemia is fourfold: (1) Determine the level of arterial obstruction and reconstitution; (2) Determine whether the occlusion is embolic or thrombotic; (3) Assist in finding the source of embolus. The most common source of emboli by far is the left heart, due to left atrial or ventricular dilation, dysrhythmia, valvular heart disease, left ventricular aneurysm, or rarely left heart tumor; for this reason, echocardiography is often indicated. Angiography can sometimes localize the source of noncardiac emboli, which can originate from aneurysms or ulcerated plaque in the aortoiliac vessels; (4) In selected cases, reopen the artery.

Treatment is chosen based upon the presumed cause, the severity of the symptoms, and the patient's clinical condition. Acute embolization is treated with surgical embolectomy or bypass grafting if the limb appears severely threatened. Thrombolytic therapy can reduce the thrombus burden, but it can be ineffective in lysing the embolic nidus itself, which is composed of organized thrombus or plaque material. Ultimately, the embolic source must be treated to prevent recurrence.

Notes

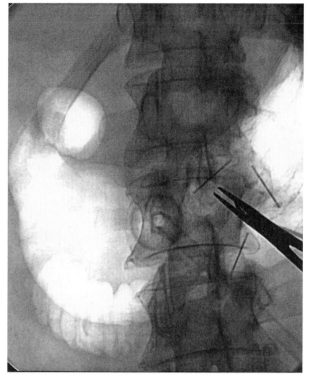

Courtesy of Dr. Daniel Brown.

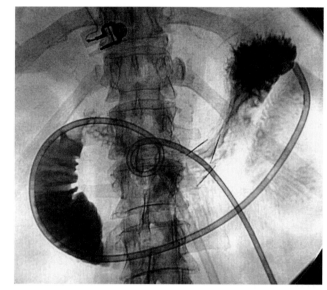

Courtesy of Dr. Daniel Brown.

1. What procedure has been performed?

2. What do the three short linear opacities overlying the gastric body represent?

3. On average, is this procedure technically more challenging than percutaneous gastrostomy tube placement?

4. Is the frequency of catheter occlusion equal to that associated with percutaneous gastrostomy tubes?

Percutaneous Gastrojejunostomy Placement

1. Percutaneous gastrojejunostomy (GJ) tube placement.

2. Gastropexy T-fasteners.

3. Yes.

4. No. GJ tubes tend to occlude more often owing to their longer length and the smaller diameter of the jejunal lumen.

Reference

Bell SD, Carmody EA, Yeung EY, et al. Percutaneous gastrostomy and gastrojejunostomy: Additional experience in 519 procedures. *Radiology.* 1995;194: 817-820.

Cross-Reference

Vascular and Interventional Radiology: THE REQUISITES, pp 532-536.

Comment

The indications for placement of a percutaneous GJ tube (either de novo or via conversion of an existing gastrostomy tube to a GJ tube) include aspiration with gastric feeding, known severe gastroesophageal reflux, gastric outlet obstruction, and decreased gastric motility (e.g., patients with diabetic gastroparesis).

From a technical standpoint, three differences from percutaneous gastrostomy tube placement are present. First, because of the increased catheter manipulation required for GJ-tube placement, gastropexy with placement of two to four T-fasteners is strongly recommended. Second, catheterization of the duodenum can be challenging in patients with pyloric stenosis or unfavorable angulation of the initial gastrostomy tract. Third, extreme care must be used to avoid buckling a loop of catheter into the stomach during placement; this can result in loss of hard-earned access into the duodenum and can lengthen procedure time. The optimal positioning of the distal part of the tube is in the proximal jejunum beyond the ligament of Treitz.

Notes

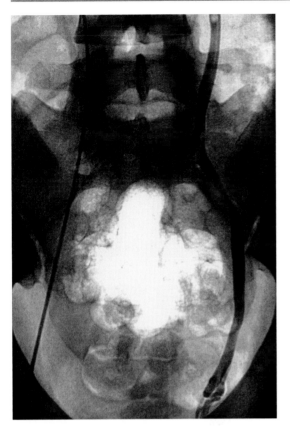
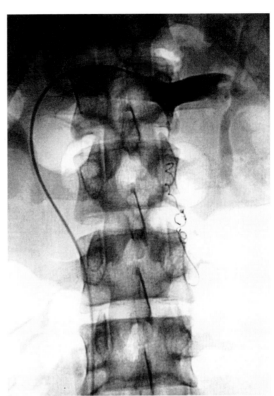

1. What vein is selectively catheterized?

2. Is this disorder more common on the left or right?

3. What are the indications for treatment?

4. What treatment options exist?

Male Varicocele

1. Left gonadal vein.

2. Left.

3. Spermatic dysfunction (male infertility), scrotal pain, scrotal enlargement or disfigurement, and testicular hypoplasia in adolescent boys.

4. Surgical ligation and percutaneous transluminal embolization.

Reference

Fretz PC, Sandlow JI. Varicocele: Current concepts in pathophysiology, diagnosis, and treatment. *Urol Clin North Am*. 2002;29:921-937.

Cross-Reference

Vascular and Interventional Radiology: THE REQUI- SITES, pp 373-374.

Comment

Varicocele is a dilation of the pampiniform plexus that affects 10% to 15% of males. Many theories have been proposed to explain primary varicocele, including abnormalities of the internal spermatic vein valves and left renal vein compression causing venous hypertension. A unilateral right varicocele or sudden onset of a varicocele in an older man should raise concern for an abdominal or pelvic mass causing venous compression and impaired venous drainage.

Most men are asymptomatic, but infertility resulting from impaired sperm motility and number, scrotal pain, and scrotal swelling and disfigurement can result. Nearly 50% of men evaluated for infertility have unilateral or bilateral varicocele. Leading theories suggest a relation to elevated scrotal temperature or reflux of metabolites from the renal and adrenal veins. Most varicoceles are detected on physical examination, but sonography, scintigraphy, and MRI are useful when the examination is normal or equivocal.

Surgical ligation and embolotherapy are the two primary treatment modalities. Embolotherapy involves performing a diagnostic venogram to confirm valvular incompetence followed by embolization of the internal spermatic vein from the level of the superior pubic ramus to the vein orifice with occlusion of collateral channels as necessary. Surgical ligation and embolotherapy demonstrate similar rates of technical success, improvement in sperm density and motility, subsequent pregnancy, and complications.

Notes

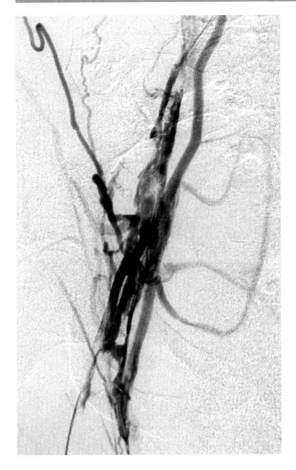 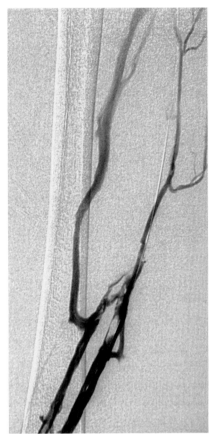

1. What type of examination has been performed?

2. What are the main clinical findings?

3. Is catheter-directed thrombolysis a good treatment option for this patient?

Chronic Deep Vein Thrombosis

1. Lower-extremity digital subtraction venogram.

2. Irregular mural filling defects, septated venous channels with surrounding collaterals, consistent with chronic deep vein thrombosis (DVT).

3. No. Thrombolysis is less likely to succeed when DVT is chronic in duration.

Reference

Prandoni P, Lensing AWA, Cogo A, et al. The long-term clinical course of acute deep-vein thrombosis. *Ann Intern Med.* 1996;125:1-7.

Cross-Reference

Vascular and Interventional Radiology: THE REQUI-SITES, pp 457-459.

Comment

From 25% to 50% of patients with deep vein thrombosis develop post-thrombotic syndrome (PTS). Patients with PTS often manifest symptoms of limb edema, aching, venous claudication, hyperpigmentation, and/or ulcerations. The symptoms are typically worse near the end of the day after the patient has been ambulatory. PTS is known to impair quality of life.

The etiology of post-thrombotic symptoms is ambulatory venous hypertension, which has two distinct components: Completed valvular damage with subsequent reflux and persistent venous obstruction due to intraluminal thrombus and debris.

Venographic findings of chronic (>2 weeks) DVT often include a septated and contracted appearance of the involved vein(s) with multiple channels, relative lack of venous dilation, and the presence of large collaterals. Sonographic findings parallel the venographic findings, and include increased echogenicity of the intraluminal material, a laminar distribution of the filling defects, and a septated appearance.

Notes

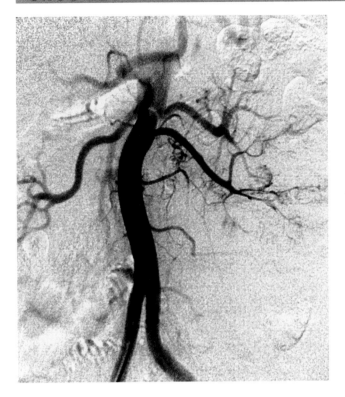

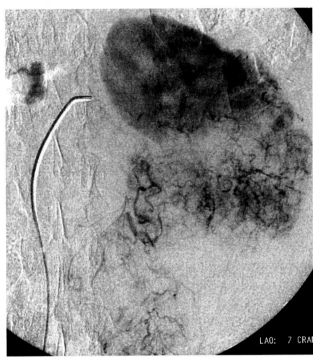

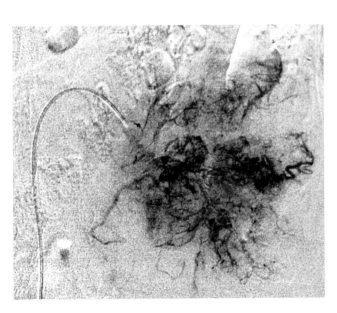

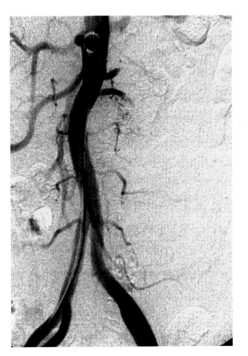

1. What is the primary angiographic finding?

2. What is the likely diagnosis?

3. What is the likely treatment for this disorder?

4. What is the role of angiography in this disorder?

Renal Cell Carcinoma

1. Large hypervascular mass replacing the lower part of the left kidney.

2. Renal cell carcinoma.

3. Radical nephrectomy (common) or partial nephrectomy (carefully selected cases).

4. Presurgical planning to determine if a partial nephrectomy will be appropriate. Also, angiography may be performed to enable preoperative embolization (as seen in the last figure), performed to diminish perioperative blood loss.

Reference

Zielinski H, Szmigielski S, Petrovich Z. Comparison of preoperative embolization followed by radical nephrectomy with radical nephrectomy alone for renal cell carcinoma. *Am J Clin Oncol.* 2000;23:6-12.

Cross-Reference

Vascular and Interventional Radiology: THE REQUISITES, pp 338-342.

Comment

Risk factors for renal cell carcinoma include tobacco use, long-term phenacetin use, von Hippel–Lindau disease (which can cause bilateral tumors), and chronic hemodialysis. Clinically, the disorder commonly manifests with gross hematuria, flank pain, and/or weight loss; less commonly, the disorder is suspected based upon the presence of a palpable mass or a paraneoplastic syndrome (hypertension, erythrocytosis, or hypercalcemia).

Imaging findings of renal cell carcinoma include a solid mass lesion on cross-sectional imaging, which can be calcified, necrotic, and/or hemorrhagic. The tumor might extend into the renal vein and/or inferior vena cava. Angiographically, 95% of tumors are hypervascular, and arteriovenous shunting and venous lakes are common. Preoperative angiographic embolization is often performed to diminish tumor vascularity and thereby reduce perioperative blood loss.

Notes

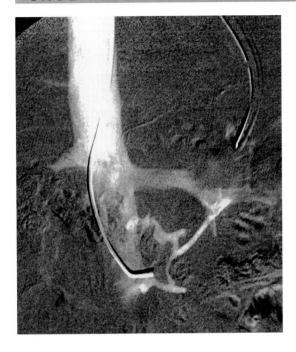

1. What anatomic variant is depicted in the first image?

2. Why is this important to diagnose when placing an inferior vena cava (IVC) filter?

3. What other venous anomalies are important to exclude before placing a filter?

4. Where should an IVC filter be?

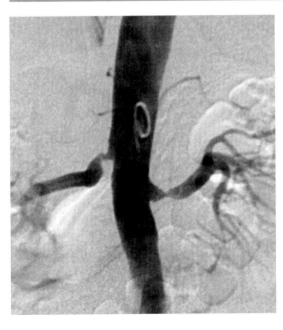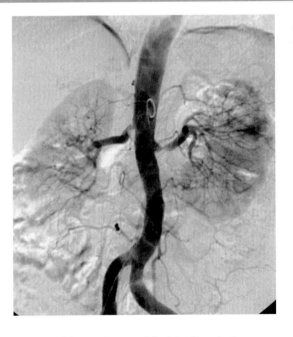

1. What are the common presenting symptoms experienced by patients with this disorder?

2. Name three potential etiologies for the lesions visualized in the images.

3. What is the most likely cause of the lesions seen in the images?

4. What treatment options are available for patients with this disorder?

CASE 49

Variant Anatomy: Circumaortic Left Renal Vein

1. Circumaortic left renal vein.

2. This segment can serve as a collateral pathway for emboli to circumvent an IVC filter and reach the lungs.

3. IVC duplication, left-sided IVC, and accessory renal veins.

4. Below the lowest renal vein if this is possible.

Reference

Trigaux JP, Vandroogenbroek S, Wilpelaere JF. Congenital anomalies of the inferior vena cava and left renal vein: Evaluation with spiral CT. *J Vasc Interv Radiol.* 1998;9:339-345.

Cross-Reference

Vascular and Interventional Radiology: THE REQUISITES, pp 350-355.

Comment

A circumaortic left renal vein is found in 1.5% to 8.7% of the population. It represents a congenital variant and results from persistence of the infrarenal segment of the left supracardinal vein. The preaortic portion of the venous ring is located in the usual position of the left renal vein. The retroaortic portion of the ring courses downward, joining the IVC in the lower lumbar region. There may be associated anomalies of drainage of the lumbar veins and left gonadal vein.

An IVC filter placed below the upper insertion but above the lower insertion of the venous ring allows the ring to serve as a potential pathway for emboli from the lower extremity or pelvis to pass up the IVC, into the lower limb of the left renal vein, and out the upper limb into the IVC above the filter. To exclude this pathway, the filter should preferably be deployed below all of the renal veins.

Accessory renal veins have a similar theoretical risk and can occur on either the right or left. As above, if possible, the IVC filter should be placed below all renal veins.

CASE 50

Atherosclerotic Renal Artery Stenosis

1. Hypertension and chronic renal failure.

2. Atherosclerosis, fibromuscular dysplasia, neurofibromatosis.

3. Atherosclerosis.

4. Aortorenal arterial bypass, percutaneous transluminal angioplasty, endovascular stent placement.

References

Gill KS, Fowler RC. Atherosclerotic renal arterial stenosis: Clinical outcomes of stent placement for hypertension and renal failure. *Radiology.* 2003;226 (3):821-826.
Olin JW. Atherosclerotic renal artery disease. *Cardiol Clin.* 2002;20:547-562.

Cross-Reference

Vascular and Interventional Radiology: THE REQUISITES, pp 327-336.

Comment

Patients with renal artery stenosis (RAS) typically present with hypertension refractory to multiple medications or chronic renal failure resulting from ischemic nephropathy. The most common cause of RAS by far is atherosclerosis. Other causes include fibromuscular dysplasia, aortic dissection, and neurofibromatosis. Atherosclerotic lesions are most commonly located in the ostial and periostial portions of the main renal artery, as in this case, but they can also be seen distally.

Surgical bypass is most commonly performed in patients with lesions not amenable to percutaneous treatment. RAS caused by atherosclerosis has a 60% to 70% patency at 5 years when treated by percutaneous balloon angioplasty; however, angioplasty of ostial lesions is associated with substantially lower patencies (25%-50%). For this reason, endovascular stents are usually used to treat ostial renal artery stenosis.

Fair Game

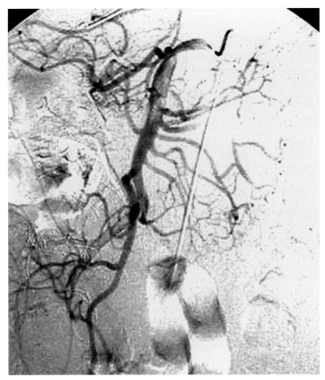

Courtesy of Dr. Thomas Vesely.

1. Specify the examination that is represented on the image above.

2. What is the major finding?

3. What is the probable etiology of this abnormality?

4. Does this abnormality need to be treated and how?

Superior Mesenteric Artery Embolus

1. Selective superior mesenteric arteriogram (SMA).

2. Globular filling defect in the proximal superior mesenteric artery.

3. Embolus from a cardiac source.

4. Yes, by emergent surgical thrombectomy.

Reference
Lee R, Tung HK, Tung PH, et al. CT in acute mesenteric ischemia. *Clin Radiol*. 2003;58:279-287.

Cross-Reference
Vascular and Interventional Radiology: THE REQUI-SITES, pp 294-296.

Comment
The image clearly demonstrates partial occlusion of the superior mesenteric artery by a globular filling defect, consistent with an embolus. The remaining SMA branches have a normal appearance.

Acute mesenteric ischemia is associated with a mortality rate of 70%, primarily due to bowel infarction with resultant sepsis. The clinical signs of mesenteric ischemia can include abdominal pain, leukocytosis, hematochezia, and lactic acidosis. Unfortunately, the clinical signs of this disorder are insidious and are often recognized after irreversible bowel ischemia has occurred. Prompt diagnosis and therapy are absolutely imperative in avoiding mortality. The etiologies of acute mesenteric ischemia include embolus (which produces ischemia within a major mesenteric vascular distribution), hypotension in patients with preexisting atherosclerotic stenoses (which can produce ischemia within a watershed distribution, usually near the splenic flexure, which represents the junction of the superior and inferior mesenteric artery territories), and acute aortic dissection.

Surgical therapy, specifically thrombectomy and/or aortomesenteric bypass with bowel resection as needed, is the treatment of choice. Endovascular methods can be used in rare cases where the embolus involves an extremely short segment near the origin of the SMA (enabling the stent to be placed), but stenting has not been shown to be equivalent to surgical therapy in this clinical setting. The special subset of patients with aortic dissection complicated by mesenteric ischemia may also be treated in endovascular fashion, using stent placement and/or percutaneous balloon fenestration of the aortic flap.

Notes

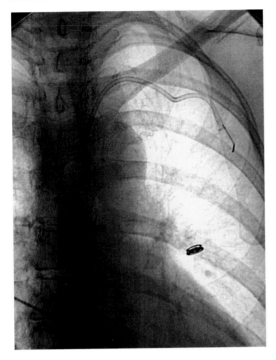
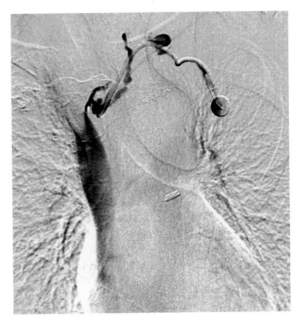

1. Where is the tip of the left-sided catheter in these images located?

2. Where should the tip be located?

3. What complication is observed in the second image?

4. Name three other complications of central venous catheter placement.

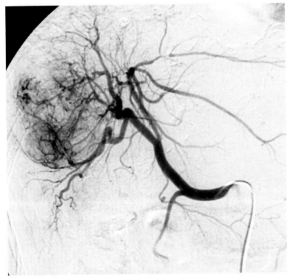
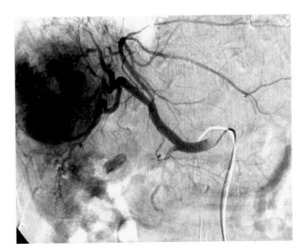

Courtesy of Dr. Daniel Brown.

Courtesy of Dr. Daniel Brown.

1. What abnormalities are apparent on this selective right hepatic arteriogram?

2. What is the most likely diagnosis?

3. What serum marker is commonly elevated in these patients?

4. What percutaneous treatments are available for this disorder?

CASE 52

Central Venous Catheter Malposition with Thrombosis

1. Left brachiocephalic vein.

2. Distal superior vena cava.

3. Thrombosis of the left brachiocephalic vein.

4. Infection with or without bacteremia, bleeding after placement, pneumothorax after placement (rare with radiologically guided placement).

Reference

Vesely TM. Central venous catheter tip position: A continuing controversy. *J Vasc Intervent Radiol.* 2003;14: 527-534.

Cross-Reference

Vascular and Interventional Radiology: THE REQUISITES, pp 180-183.

Comment

Radiologists can place the entire gamut of central venous catheters: (1) Peripherally inserted central catheters (PICC lines): These small-caliber catheters are used for short-term (2-6 weeks) venous access and are inserted via an arm vein; (2) Nontunneled or tunneled (for long-term access) catheters for administering blood transfusions, antibiotics, other parenteral medications, and/or total parenteral nutrition; (3) Nontunneled or tunneled pheresis catheters; (4) Nontunneled or tunneled hemodialysis catheters; (5) Implantable ports for intermittent access.

In general, the internal jugular (IJ) vein is the preferred approach for placing tunneled (long-term) catheters and ports. The IJ approach is associated with a lower incidence of catheter migration, pinch-off syndrome, and symptomatic venous occlusion. Furthermore, IJ access spares the subclavian veins; this is extremely important in patients with chronic renal failure for whom upper extremity dialysis access might eventually be needed. For nontunneled catheters, the subclavian vein is generally preferred because chest wall exit sites are associated with a lower infection rate than neck or groin exit sites. However, notable exceptions to this rule include the aforementioned patients with chronic renal failure and those with impaired coagulation, because the subclavian vein is located in a less-compressible location than the IJ.

Although most organizational guidelines recommend placing the catheter tip in the distal superior vena cava, a significant number of physicians are placing hemodialysis and pheresis catheters in the proximal right atrium in order to achieve better flow rates.

CASE 53

Hepatocellular Carcinoma

1. Hypervascularity, neovascularity, splaying of arterial branches, dense tumor stain.

2. Hepatocellular carcinoma.

3. Alpha-fetoprotein.

4. Embolization with bland particles and/or chemotherapeutic agents, radioembolization with yttrium-90, hepatic arterial port catheter insertion for chemotherapy, percutaneous ethanol ablation, radiofrequency ablation, and cryoablation.

Reference

Sze DY, Razavi MK, So SK, et al. Impact of multidetector CT hepatic arteriography on the planning of chemoembolization treatment of hepatocellular carcinoma. *AJR Am J Roentgenol.* 2001;177:1339-1345.

Cross-Reference

Vascular and Interventional Radiology: THE REQUISITES, pp 306-308.

Comment

Hepatocellular carcinoma can manifest with a solitary mass, multiple masses, or diffuse hepatic involvement. Commonly found in patients with cirrhosis, it is a highly malignant neoplasm with a poor long-term prognosis. Angiographic features include enlarged feeding arteries, neovascularity, puddling, dense tumor stain, arterioportal shunting, portal vein invasion, and occasionally hepatic vein invasion. A central necrotic area may be present and can splay surrounding abnormal vessels. The uninvolved liver commonly shows arteriographic changes of cirrhosis, including small corkscrew-like vessels.

Arteriography is useful for assessing tumor blood supply before surgery and for providing guidance for hepatic arterial port catheter placement or chemoembolization. It is useful to obtain portal venous images at the time of arteriography to determine the direction of portal venous flow and to detect thrombus in the portal vein.

Because hepatocellular carcinomas derive their blood supply nearly entirely from the hepatic arterial system, they are significantly more sensitive to the ischemic effects of arterial occlusion than normal hepatic parenchyma, which derives more than two thirds of its blood supply from the portal venous system. Chemoembolization, which involves intraarterial infusion of chemotherapy immediately followed by embolization, results in two important effects that constitute the basis for this form of therapy: increased dwell time of the chemotherapeutic agents within the tumor owing to slow flow in and out of the tumor bed, and tumor ischemia.

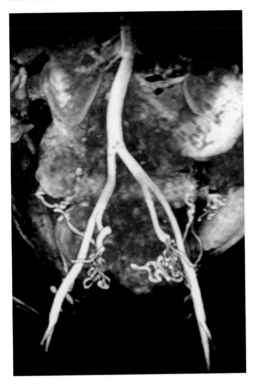
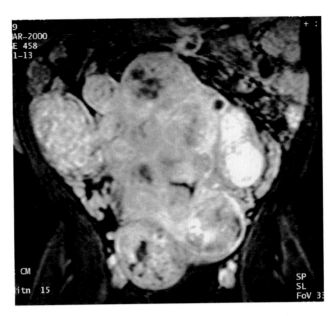

1. What study is presented in the images above?

2. Why was this study requested by the interventional radiologist?

3. What common cause of global uterine enlargement may be distinguished from uterine fibroid disease using this study?

4. What common arterial variants can this study help to identify?

Enlarged Uterine Arteries

1. Magnetic resonance angiogram (MRA) of the uterine arteries.

2. Planning for uterine fibroid embolization (UFE).

3. Adenomyosis.

4. Unilateral absence of the uterine artery, ovarian artery supply to the uterus.

Reference

Spies JB, Roth AR, Jha RC, et al. Leiomyomata treated with uterine artery embolization: Factors associated with successful symptom and imaging outcome. *Radiology*. 2002;222:45-52.

Cross-Reference

Vascular and Interventional Radiology: THE REQUI-SITES, pp 208-282.

Comment

The first image demonstrates the characteristic tortuous appearance of enlarged uterine arteries as they descend into the pelvis and then ascend along the lateral uterine wall. The second image demonstrates strong heterogeneous enhancement of the uterus and the individual fibroid tumors on MRI following gadolinium infusion, a typical appearance.

MRI is useful in the preembolization workup of patients with uterine fibroids for several reasons: (1) MRI is extremely accurate in diagnosing uterine fibroids and can distinguish between the diverse causes of global uterine enlargement: (2) MRI can accurately depict the local invasiveness of a mass lesion (triggering suspicion for malignancy); (3) MRI enables accurate and reproducible measurements to be obtained; (4) MRI can accurately classify fibroids as being submucosal, intramural, subserosal, and/or pedunculated. This information can affect the type of therapy employed; (5) Speculated causes of clinical failure of UFE include aberrant uterine artery anatomy, untreated ovarian artery supply to fibroids, and coexistent adenomyosis, all of which can be identified by MRI.

Other MRI findings might also soon be used to predict treatment response to UFE. In recent studies, submucosal fibroid location, small fibroid size, low T1 signal, and hypervascularity have been correlated with greater fibroid volume reduction after UFE, and high T1 signal has been correlated with lesser volume reductions. Hence, although ultrasound is an acceptable diagnostic modality for fibroids, interventional radiologists are increasingly turning to MRI for its superior pretreatment planning capabilities.

Notes

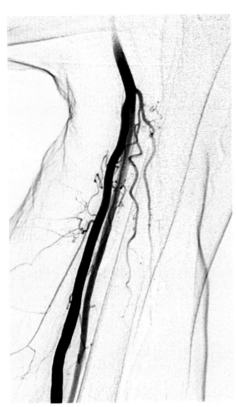

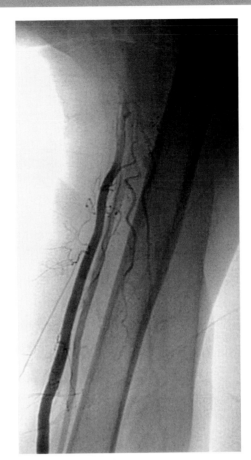

Courtesy of Dr. Daniel Brown.   *Courtesy of Dr. Daniel Brown.*

1. Name the more medial artery on the left arm images above.

2. Name the more lateral artery on the left arm images above.

3. What symptoms are typically associated with this finding?

4. Where does the more lateral artery normally arise?

CASE 55

Variant Anatomy: High Radial Artery Origin

1. Left brachial artery.

2. Left radial artery (high origin).

3. None.

4. From the brachial artery below the elbow joint.

Reference

Uglietta JP, Kadir S. Arteriographic study of variant arterial anatomy of the upper extremities. *Cardiovasc Intervent Radiol.* 1989;12(3):145-148.

Cross-Reference

Vascular and Interventional Radiology: THE REQUISITES, pp 142-145.

Comment

Distal to the elbow joint, the brachial artery normally trifurcates into a radial artery, an ulnar artery, and an interosseous artery. Several anatomic variants of this pattern occur with enough frequency that it is important to be aware of them. For instance, in some patients the brachial artery divides proximally into two limbs that continue in parallel, then reunite distally.

Normally the radial artery arises as the first branch of the brachial artery below the elbow, and the ulnar artery divides into its named branches a few centimeters distally. However, up to 19% of persons have an early bifurcation of the brachial artery, an anomaly more commonly found on the right. Although a high radial artery origin from the brachial artery is the most common upper-extremity arterial variant (7%–8%), the ulnar artery can also arise from the brachial artery above the elbow. Less commonly, the radial artery (1%–3%) or ulnar artery (1%–2%) can arise from the axillary artery. Physiologically these variations are of little significance, but they can be significant when a brachial artery puncture is planned or when a patient suffers trauma to the upper extremity with associated vascular injury.

Notes

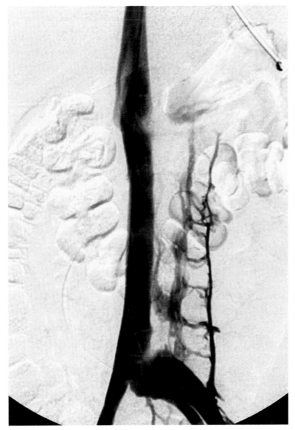

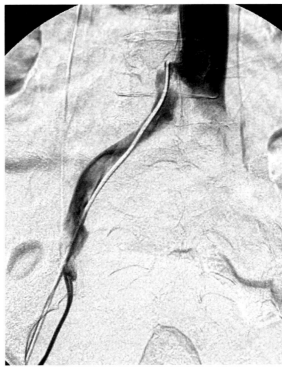

Courtesy of Dr. James Duncan.

Courtesy of Dr. James Duncan.

1. What findings are present in these two patients and what syndrome is present in the second patient?

2. What is thought to be the etiology of this disorder?

3. What is currently favored as the treatment of choice for this disorder?

4. What is the post-thrombotic syndrome?

May–Thurner Syndrome

1. Both patients have left common iliac vein stenosis. The second patient has left iliofemoral venous thrombosis, consistent with iliac vein compression (May–Thurner) syndrome.

2. Compression of the left iliac vein by the crossing right common iliac artery.

3. Catheter-directed thrombolysis followed by iliac vein stent placement.

4. The major long-term complication of deep vein thrombosis (DVT), characterized by chronic edema, pain, skin discoloration, varicosities, venous claudication, venous stasis ulcers, and subcutaneous fibrosis.

Reference

Patel NH, Stookey KR, Ketcham DB, et al. Endovascular management of acute extensive iliofemoral deep venous thrombosis caused by May–Thurner syndrome. *J Vasc Intervent Radiol.* 2000;11:1297-1302.

Cross-Reference

Vascular and Interventional Radiology: THE REQUISITES, pp 452-457.

Comment

Iliofemoral deep venous thrombosis is three to eight times more common in the left leg than in the right leg. This is thought to be due to the relative compression of the left iliac vein at the pelvic brim by the crossing right common iliac artery.

Iliac vein compression (May–Thurner syndrome) is a distinct entity that typically affects women in the second to fourth decades. It is differentiated from bland deep vein thrombosis of the lower extremity by the presence of a fibrous spur or adhesion in the left common iliac vein, thought to represent an inflammatory response to chronic compression of the vein and irritation of its endothelium from adjacent arterial pulsations.

Patients typically present with acute iliofemoral DVT or chronic DVT with venous insufficiency. Endovascular therapy is the treatment of choice for this disorder. Typically, catheter-directed thrombolysis is used first to remove any acute thrombus, and an endovascular stent is subsequently placed to address the venous stenosis. Surgical thrombectomy that does not also address the underlying left common iliac vein stenosis has a high failure rate.

Notes

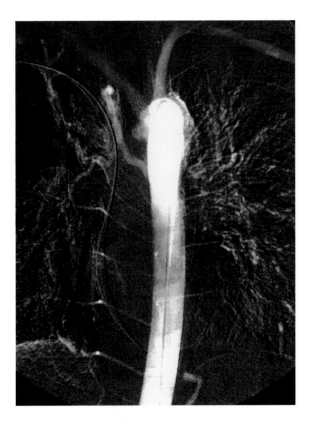 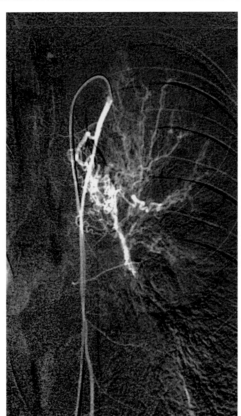

1. What abnormality is seen in the first image?

2. How did this patient likely present?

3. What are the most common causes?

4. How and why was the second image obtained?

Bronchial Artery Embolization

1. Enlarged right bronchial artery.

2. Massive hemoptysis.

3. In the non-Western world: pulmonary tuberculosis. In the Western world: cystic fibrosis, bronchogenic carcinoma, bronchiectasis, or aspergillosis.

4. Selective angiography of the left internal mammary artery was performed because this vessel is a common source of systemic collateral supply to the lungs.

Reference

Yoon W, Kim JK, Kim YH, et al. Bronchial and nonbronchial systemic artery embolization for life-threatening hemoptysis: A comprehensive review. *Radiographics.* 2002;22:1395-1409.

Cross-Reference

Vascular and Interventional Radiology: THE REQUISITES, pp 215-217.

Comment

Bronchial artery embolization has become an established procedure for treating life-threatening hemoptysis. Massive hemoptysis is usually defined by the production of 300 to 600 mL of blood per day, but the patient's clinical condition should guide therapy because smaller amounts of bleeding can be life-threatening in some instances.

In 90% of patients, bleeding arises from a bronchial artery. Less-common sources include the pulmonary arteries, aorta, and systemic collaterals to the lungs. Localization of the bleeding site by radiography, bronchoscopy, and/or chest CT before angiography and embolization is important so as to focus therapy. Hypertrophied and tortuous bronchial arteries, neovascularity, hypervascularity, and pulmonary arteriovenous shunting are common angiographic findings. Extravasation of contrast is rarely seen.

The bronchial arteries typically originate from the descending thoracic aorta at the T5-T6 level. In about 40% of patients, there are two arteries on the left and one on the right arising from an intercostobronchial trunk. However, there is extensive variability in number, origin, and branching pattern. It is very important to identify spinal arterial branches that arise from the bronchial and intercostal arteries, because nontarget embolization of these vessels can result in spinal ischemia. In general, embolization with polyvinyl alcohol particles is preferred. Coils are not used because they produce proximal occlusion, precluding repeat embolization should hemoptysis recur.

Notes

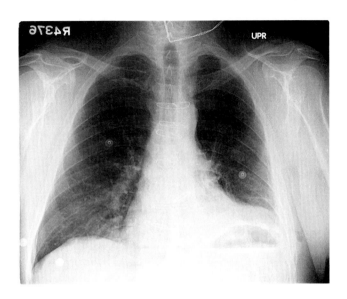 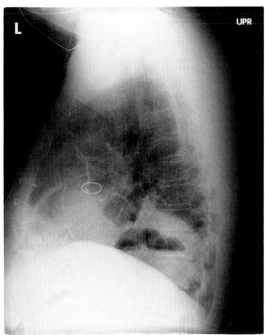

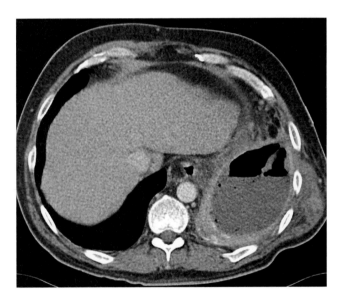 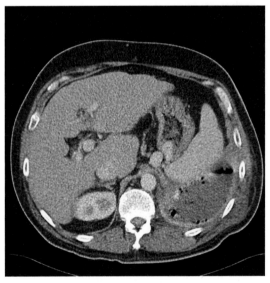

1. What is the primary abnormality?

2. What symptoms are likely present?

3. What is the best initial invasive treatment option for this patient?

4. If catheter placement did not result in adequate drainage, what adjunctive therapy could be performed?

Empyema

1. Left posterior empyema.

2. Fever, leukocytosis, pleuritic chest pain, and possibly dyspnea and/or sepsis.

3. Percutaneous thoracostomy.

4. Intracavitary infusion of a fibrinolytic agent.

Reference

VanSonnenberg E, Wittich GR, Goodacre BW, et al. Percutaneous drainage of thoracic collections. *J Thorac Imaging.* 1998;13:(2)74-82.

Cross-Reference

Vascular and Interventional Radiology: THE REQUISITES, pp 516-518.

Comment

The images demonstrate a rim-enhancing, gas-containing fluid collection within the left posterior pleural space, consistent with empyema. Imaging-guided chest tube placement is an excellent initial therapy and can be performed under fluoroscopy, CT, or ultrasound guidance. Preprocedural clinical assessment should include an evaluation of whether the patient will be able to tolerate the required position on the procedure table, because many patients with empyema have significant associated pulmonary compromise. Coagulation studies and platelet level should also be obtained.

Under imaging guidance, a needle is placed into the collection and contrast is injected to confirm proper positioning. It is important to avoid placing the needle just under a rib, because this can result in hemorrhage due to traversal of an intercostal artery. Over a guidewire, the tract is dilated and a large-bore drainage catheter is placed and attached to negative pressure. Follow-up CT scans are used to evaluate the progress of drainage. When the patient has improved clinically and the cavity is resolved, the catheter can be incrementally withdrawn to allow gradual healing of the residual cavity and tube tract.

If drainage ceases or stabilizes before the collection completely resolves, the cavity may be loculated and intracavitary fibrinolytic agents can be given. Alternatively, the catheter might be occluded or might not be in optimal position; a repeat CT scan can be used to guide an attempt at repositioning the catheter under fluoroscopy. If the catheter is patent and in optimal position, then a larger catheter may be needed. Infrequently, the fluid may simply be too viscous for percutaneous drainage, and surgery may be required.

Notes

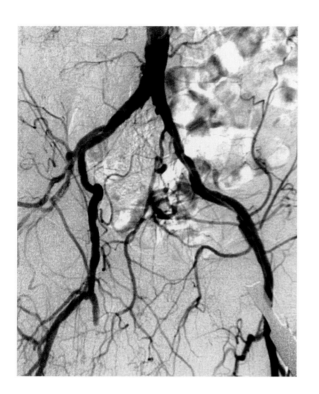
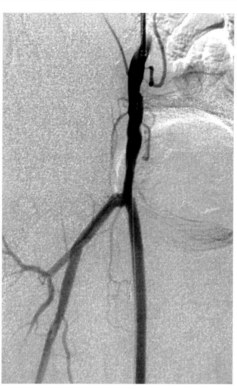
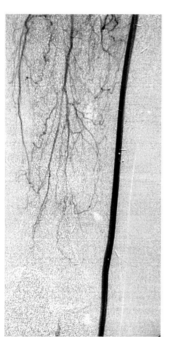
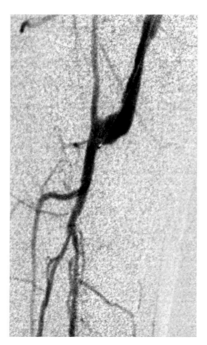

1. What vascular problem is present in the first image?

2. What are the common causes of this problem?

3. What intervention was performed between the first two images?

4. What are the two most feared complications of endovascular intervention in the treatment of this problem?

Bypass Graft Occlusion and Thrombolysis

1. Occlusion of a bypass graft originating in the right common femoral artery.

2. Proximal or distal anastomotic stenosis, intragraft stenosis, progression of atherosclerosis proximal or distal to the graft, hypercoagulability, and mechanical compression.

3. Catheter-directed thrombolysis or surgical thrombectomy.

4. Distant hemorrhage and distal embolization of thrombus.

Reference

Ouriel K. Current status of thrombolysis for peripheral arterial occlusive disease. *Ann Vasc Surg.* 2002;16: 797-804.

Cross-Reference

Vascular and Interventional Radiology: THE REQUI-SITES, pp 429-433.

Comment

The first image demonstrates the stump of an occluded right femoropopliteal artery bypass graft. Graft occlusion is commonly the result of stenosis at the anastomosic sites.

The precise role of thrombolysis in the treatment of bypass graft thrombosis is somewhat controversial. However, several published trials support its use for patients with acute (<2 weeks) graft occlusion to achieve the following benefits: (1) It avoids surgical risks in patients who often have vascular comorbidities; (2) It has potential to both declot the graft and treat an underlying stenosis using angioplasty or stent placement; (3) Even if treatment of the underlying disorder cannot be achieved percutaneously, the diagnostic information provided by angiography after thrombolysis often guides definitive surgical therapy and enables reduction of the planned level of surgery. Endovascular therapy tends to be more successful in treating occluded synthetic grafts compared with vein grafts.

Disadvantages of thrombolysis include the longer time to reperfusion compared with surgical thrombectomy, and the risk of complications. Approximately 10% of patients require a transfusion due to bleeding, which most commonly occurs at the arterial access site. Distant bleeding occurs in 1% to 2% of patients, and intracranial bleeding occurs in 0.5% to 1.0%. Distal embolization occurs in 5% to 12% of patients, but it is usually treatable and rarely results in amputation. Compartment syndrome occurs in 2% of patients.

Notes

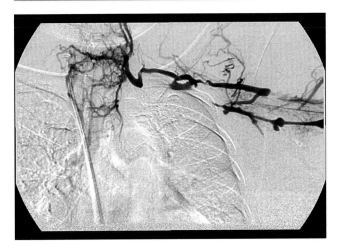

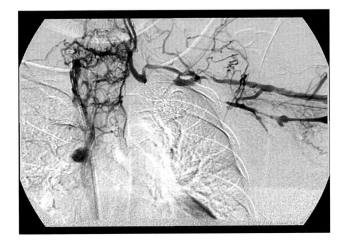

1. What abnormality is present on the images?

2. What is the most common cause of this problem?

3. How long have this patient's symptoms likely been present?

4. Should endovascular treatment be performed?

Chronic Axillosubclavian Vein Occlusion

1. Left axillosubclavian vein occlusion.

2. Central venous catheters and pacemakers.

3. More than 2 weeks.

4. No.

Reference

Meissner MH. Axillary-subclavian venous thrombosis. *Rev Cardiovasc Med.* 2002;3(Suppl 2):S44-S51.

Cross-Reference

Vascular and Interventional Radiology: THE REQUI-SITES, pp 168-173.

Comment

The images demonstrate occlusion of the left axillo-subclavian vein with collateral reconstitution of the superior vena cava. Venographic features that strongly suggest a chronic process include the lack of significant dilation of the occluded veins, the somewhat tapered aspect of the occlusion, the lack of globular filling defects or a meniscus sign, and the presence of abundant collaterals.

Most patients with subclavian vein thrombosis experience initial upper-extremity swelling and/or pain, but these symptoms usually subside as a mature venous collateral network develops. In fact, about 80% of patients with subclavian vein thrombosis eventually become asymptomatic or minimally symptomatic with antico-agulation therapy alone. For these reasons, endovascular interventions to restore patency in patients with subcla-vian vein thrombosis are reserved for carefully selected patients with primary axillosubclavian thrombosis (i.e., due to thoracic outlet syndrome), for young patients with acute secondary subclavian venous thrombosis who have good functional status, and for rare patients with special concerns such as a continuing need for central venous access where no other access sites are available. In these patients, a trial of thrombolytic therapy may be used, but most patients with chronic secondary subclavian vein thrombosis are treated with anticoagulation and removal of any central venous catheter that is present in the thrombus-containing vein.

Notes

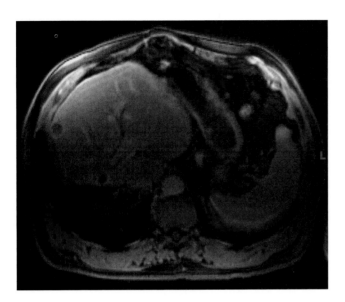 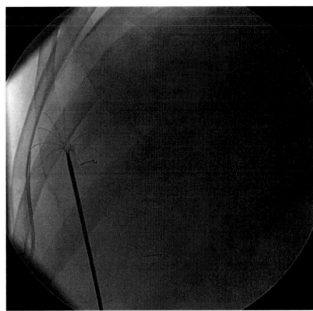

1. What is the abnormality in the first image?

2. What procedure is being performed in the second image?

3. What potential complication can this patient develop based on the anatomic location of the lesion?

4. What adjunctive measure was performed in the second image to avoid this complication?

Liver Metastasis: Radiofrequency Ablation

1. Metastatic liver lesion (from colorectal carcinoma).

2. Radiofrequency ablation (RFA).

3. Thermal injury to the diaphragm.

4. An angiographic catheter has been interposed between the liver surface and the diaphragm; it was used to instill saline during the ablation procedure.

Reference

McGhana JP, Dodd 3rd GD. Radiofrequency ablation of the liver: Current status. *AJR Am J Roentgenol.* 2001; 176:3-16.

Cross-Reference

Vascular and Interventional Radiology: THE REQUISITES, pp 674-681.

Comment

Surgical resection remains the standard of care for metastatic liver lesions; however, only 5% to 15% of patients are eligible for resection. RFA of nonresectable lesions can be performed in a subset of this patient population. Generally accepted selection criteria include fewer than five lesions, each less than 5 cm in diameter, and no extrahepatic disease. Anatomic factors that must be taken into consideration include the location of the tumor(s) in relation to intrahepatic structures such as the bile ducts and vessels. Large vessels in close proximity to the lesion can make it difficult to attain good ablation due to a heat sink effect: Relatively high blood flow rates cause a cooling effect on the adjacent tissue. Extrahepatic structures such as the gallbladder, diaphragm, and adjacent bowel should also be evaluated for proximity to the anticipated ablation zone to prevent thermal injury to these structures.

The mechanism of action is the transmission of radiofrequency waves to the tissues, which causes an elevation of tissue temperature leading to coagulative necrosis of the exposed tissues. Image guidance by US, CT, or even MRI is used for correct needle placement through a percutaneous approach. The procedure can be performed under moderate sedation or general anesthesia. Certain adjunctive procedures can be performed to create a safe zone between the lesion and adjacent structures to prevent thermal injury, including patient positioning and hydrodissection (as in this case). Combination therapy with transarterial chemoembolization may also be performed.

Notes

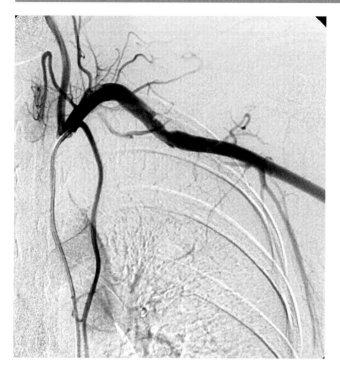

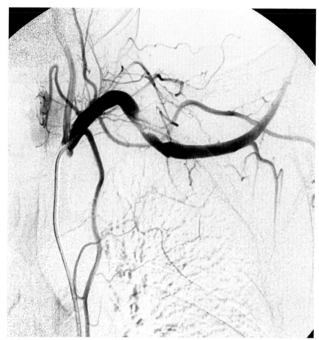

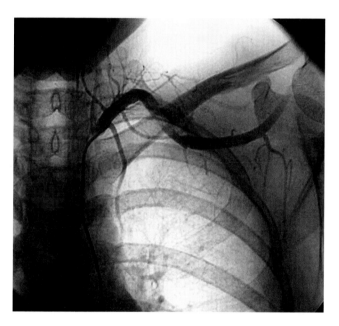

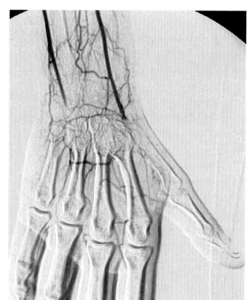

1. What positioning maneuver would worsen the abnormality in the first image?

2. What finding in the third image provides an important clue to the diagnosis?

3. What complication has this patient developed?

4. How would this be treated?

Arterial Thoracic Outlet Compression Syndrome

1. Abduction at the shoulder joint.

2. A cervical rib.

3. Distal embolization of thrombus.

4. Surgical thoracic outlet decompression with embolectomy.

Reference

Demondion X, Bacqueville E, Paul C, et al. Thoracic outlet: assessment with MR imaging in asymptomatic and symptomatic populations. *Radiology*. 2003;227: 461-468.

Cross-Reference

Vascular and Interventional Radiology: THE REQUISITES, pp 154-155.

Comment

Patients with arterial thoracic outlet compression syndrome typically present with symptoms in the hand and fingers including pain, numbness, paresthesias, intermittent claudication, cool skin temperature, and occasionally severe digital ischemia. Nearly half exhibit symptoms of Raynaud's phenomenon. Symptoms often worsen with arm abduction. Reduction or obliteration of the radial pulse during clinical maneuvers such as passive arm hyperabduction or Adson's maneuver (deep inspiration with hyperextension of the neck while the head is rotated to the symptomatic side) are highly suggestive of the diagnosis. A systolic bruit can sometimes be heard at the site of compression.

Cervical ribs are present in up to 0.5% of persons in the general population, but less than half of these patients develop symptoms of neurovascular compression. However, of patients with thoracic outlet compression syndrome, about 70% have a cervical rib. Other problems that can result in compression include the presence of a scalenus minimus muscle (seen in one third of normal persons), a wide or abnormal insertion or enlargement of the anterior scalene muscle, an anomalous first rib narrowing of the costoclavicular space, healed fracture deformities of the clavicle or first rib, or a muscular body habitus narrowing the pectoralis minor tunnel.

Arteriography should be performed with selective subclavian artery injection in a neutral position and with passive abduction of the extremity. Arteriographic findings include subclavian artery compression or narrowing with or without post-stenotic dilation, arterial occlusion, aneurysm, mural thrombus formation, and/or distal embolization.

Notes

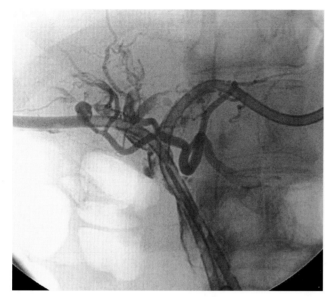

Courtesy of Dr. Daniel Brown.

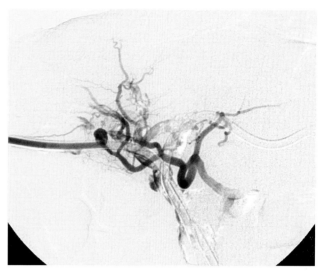

Courtesy of Dr. Daniel Brown.

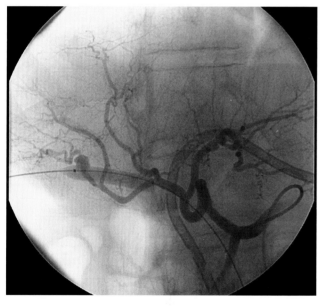

Courtesy of Dr. Daniel Brown.

1. How did this patient probably present and how commonly does this occur?

2. What is the diagnosis?

3. What was done between the second and third images?

4. Name another major complication that can occur following percutaneous transhepatic cholangiography (PTC) and percutaneous biliary drainage (PBD)?

Iatrogenic Hepatic Artery Pseudoaneurysm

1. Hemobilia. This occurs in 2% to 10% of PTC and PBD procedures.

2. Iatrogenic pseudoaneurysm of a right hepatic artery branch.

3. The catheter was withdrawn over a wire and an angioplasty balloon catheter was inflated at the site of the pseudoaneurysm.

4. Biliary infection in the form of fever or chills, septicemia, and/or cholangitis.

Reference

Winick AB, Waybill PN, Venbrux AC. Complications of percutaneous transhepatic biliary interventions. *Tech Vasc Intervent Radiol.* 2001;4(3):200-206.

Cross-Reference

Vascular and Interventional Radiology: THE REQUISITES, pp 574-577.

Comment

Hemobilia following PTC or PBD can be a life-threatening condition, and patients should be instructed to contact the interventional radiologist immediately if they note bloody output from the drainage tube or skin site. Most bleeding, resulting from a catheter side hole within the liver parenchyma or a transient fistula between a bile duct and a portal or hepatic vein branch, is transient and resolves with conservative management. Catheter repositioning or upsizing may be necessary in some of these cases.

Severe hemobilia is usually the result of a bile duct communication with a hepatic artery branch or a major venous branch. Arterial bleeding should be suspected when pulsatile bright red blood drains from the biliary drainage catheter; in these cases, emergent hepatic arteriography is indicated for further evaluation. If arteriography does not demonstrate a site of bleeding, the biliary drainage catheter should be removed over a guidewire and the angiogram should be repeated. A balloon catheter can be replaced to tamponade bleeding while the bleeding vessel is embolized. A variety of embolic agents can be used in this setting, but most interventionalists use coils for this indication. When performing coil embolization of a pseudoaneurysm, it is important to place coils distal to, across, and proximal to the entry site to the pseudoaneurysm sac to prevent recurrent hemorrhage due to backbleeding from peripheral arterial branches.

Notes

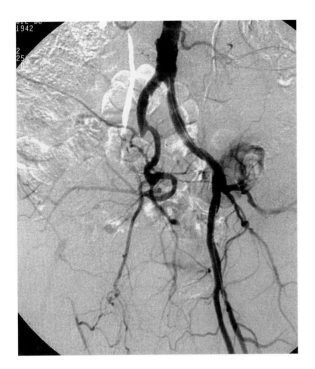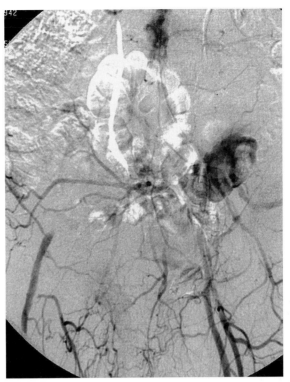

1. Describe the findings on the images above.

2. What treatment options are available?

3. If the right superficial femoral artery is also occluded, what symptom would likely be present?

4. If the right superficial femoral artery is also occluded, what therapy is indicated?

C A S E 6 4

Iliac Artery Occlusion (Atherosclerosis)

1. Right external iliac artery occlusion with common femoral artery reconstitution.

2. Aortofemoral bypass, femorofemoral bypass, thrombolysis and stent placement.

3. Rest pain.

4. Inflow reconstruction, probably via surgical bypass, is performed first. The patient is reassessed, and if lifestyle-limiting symptoms are still present, then femoropopliteal or femoral–distal bypass could be considered.

Reference

Rzucidlo EM, Powell RJ, Zwolak RM, et al. Early results of stent-grafting to treat diffuse aortoiliac occlusive disease. *J Vasc Surg*. 2003;37:1175-1180.

Cross-Reference

Vascular and Interventional Radiology: THE REQUI-SITES, pp 261-270.

Comment

The first image demonstrates an occluded right external iliac artery due to in situ thrombosis of an atherosclerotic stenosis. The second image demonstrates reconstitution of the common femoral artery, information that is critical in planning revascularization.

Aortofemoral bypass is associated with 90% patency at 5 years. In patients who have a normal contralateral iliac artery and in whom medical comorbidities are present, femorofemoral bypass is sometimes used to revascularize the ischemic limb.

Endovascular recanalization of the occluded iliac artery has been performed for many years. In patients with chronic occlusions and short-segment acute occlusions, primary stent placement is considered by many to be the optimal endovascular method. In patients with acute occlusions with longer segments of thrombus, an initial course of thrombolytic therapy is favored by most physicians to eliminate as much thrombus as possible and thereby prevent embolization during later stent placement. Hence, in contrast to iliac artery stenoses, iliac artery occlusions are usually not treated with angioplasty alone; stents are nearly always used. Although stent-based endovascular recanalization is associated with lower primary patency than surgical bypass, the secondary patency (patency with repeat interventions) is comparable to surgical bypass and the overall procedural morbidity is lower. In recent years, stent grafts have shown promise as a way to recanalize the occluded iliac artery with a lower potential for late restenosis.

Notes

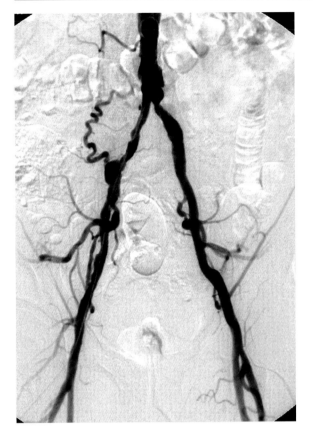 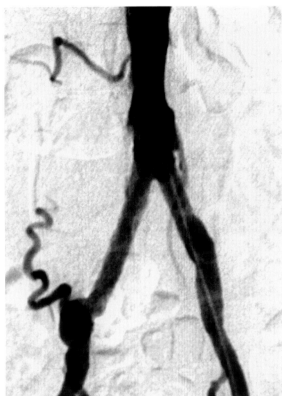

1. If the infrainguinal arteries are normal, what symptoms would this patient have?

2. Describe the angiographic findings in the first image.

3. What options are there for treatment?

4. What intervention was performed (second image) and why?

Bilateral Common Iliac Artery Stenoses (Kissing Stents)

1. Bilateral hip and buttock claudication, possibly with impotence.

2. Bilateral common iliac artery stenoses, prominent right-sided lumbar collateral.

3. Percutaneous transluminal angioplasty, stent placement, aortobifemoral bypass.

4. Kissing stents were placed. Percutaneous intervention was chosen because of its lower morbidity than surgical therapy. Stenting was chosen over angioplasty because of the eccentric nature of the right-sided stenosis. Kissing stents were placed because of the involvement of the aortoiliac junction.

Reference

Scheinert D, Schroder M, Balzer JO, et al. Stent-supported reconstruction of the aortoiliac bifurcation with the kissing balloon technique. *Circulation*. 1999;100(Suppl 19):II295-II300.

Cross-Reference

Vascular and Interventional Radiology: THE REQUISITES, pp 261-270.

Comment

Patients with disease in the aorta or common iliac arteries typically present with hip and buttock claudication and/or impotence, because of limited flow into the internal iliac artery territories. Intermittent claudication generally occurs when ankle–brachial indices are 0.5 to 0.9. When additional levels of disease are present in the femoral and/or tibial vessels, the patient is likely to experience rest pain in the feet. Rest pain signifies limb-threatening ischemia and is associated with a high amputation rate if the vascular abnormality is not treated. Ankle–brachial indices are generally 0.2 to 0.4 in patients with rest pain and no visible tissue loss, and they may be lower in patients with ulcers or gangrene.

Surgical aortofemoral bypass is associated with 90% patency at 5 years. The secondary patency of iliac artery angioplasty with selective stent placement is 80% to 90% at 4 years. Because endovascular therapy is associated with lower mortality and major morbidity, it is the preferred first-line treatment in patients with anatomically suitable iliac lesions.

Patients with aortoiliac junction lesions with or without actual distal aortic stenosis are often treated with kissing stents regardless of whether the contralateral iliac artery is diseased. This is done to effectively cover the aortic bifurcation plaque, to provide support to the other inflated balloon, and to prevent embolization down the contralateral side due to dislodged aortic bifurcation plaque.

Notes

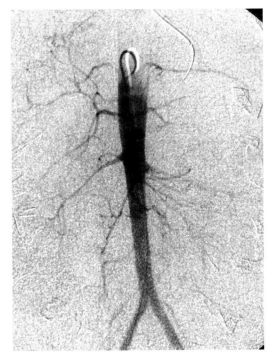
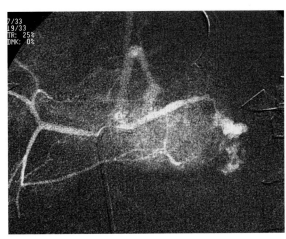

1. What vascular problem is depicted in the first image of this adult patient?

2. Describe the examination depicted in the second image.

3. What is the primary abnormality in the second image?

4. How might this problem be treated?

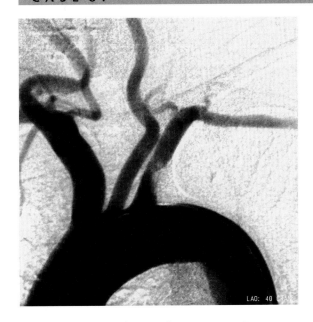

1. What vascular abnormality is present?

2. Name three clinical sequelae that can result from this lesion.

3. What finding might confound endovascular management of this lesion?

4. What is the standard treatment for this problem?

CASE 66

Traumatic Splenic Artery Injury

1. The diminutive caliber of the aortic branch vessels indicates systemic vasoconstriction due to hypovolemic shock.

2. Selective celiac arteriogram.

3. Splenic artery injury with pseudoaneurysm formation.

4. Transcatheter embolization or surgical repair.

Reference

Kluger Y, Rabau M. Improved success in nonoperative management of blunt splenic injury: Embolization of splenic artery pseudoaneurysm. *J Trauma.* 1998; 45:980-981.

Cross-Reference

Vascular and Interventional Radiology: THE REQUISITES, pp 313-314.

Comment

Angiographic findings of visceral arterial trauma can include displacement or splaying of arterial branches due to hematoma formation, pseudoaneurysms, contrast extravasation, arterial filling defects due thrombosis or dissection, and diffuse vasoconstriction due to hypovolemic shock. In the latter instance, the extremely small caliber of the visceral vessels can occasionally render selective catheterization difficult. The patient depicted in these images is in dire need of fluid and blood product resuscitation.

When evaluating the patient with abdominal trauma, a reasonable plan for identifying the bleeding artery can only be developed after reviewing an abdominal CT scan, the results of diagnostic peritoneal lavage, and surgical findings (if the patient has already been explored). Because time is of the essence, the angiographer must direct his or her attention to the most likely source of bleeding. An abdominal aortogram may be performed initially. Although this only detects the grossest forms of branch vessel hemorrhage, it can help in selecting branch vessels in patients with distorted anatomy. The visceral vessels should then be evaluated with selective arteriography, and the vessels most likely to represent the source of bleeding should be studied first.

Traditional treatment of trauma-induced splenic arterial injuries has been splenic artery ligation with splenectomy. In recent years, transcatheter embolization has evolved into a less morbid alternative that might allow the spleen to be conserved. However, because splenic infarcts occur with moderate frequency following embolization, patients should receive appropriate immunizations to prevent later episodes of bacteremia.

CASE 67

Subclavian Artery Stenosis with Adherent Thrombus

1. Left subclavian artery stenosis with adherent filling defects.

2. Distal embolization, vertebrobasilar insufficiency due to subclavian steal, left arm claudication.

3. The visualized filling defects probably represent thrombus that could embolize during catheter manipulations.

4. Carotid–subclavian artery bypass.

Reference

Rodriguez-Lopez JA, Werner A, Martinez R, et al. Stenting for atherosclerotic occlusive disease of the subclavian artery. *Ann Vasc Surg.* 1999;13(3):254-260.

Cross-Reference

Vascular and Interventional Radiology: THE REQUISITES, pp 149-151.

Comment

The image demonstrates a moderate-caliber stenosis of the proximal left subclavian artery. Associated filling defects are present that could indicate the presence of associated thrombus, versus less-likely bulky atherosclerotic plaque. Distal embolization from this lesion is a significant concern.

The standard treatment for a proximal subclavian artery lesion is carotid–subclavian artery bypass, which is associated with extremely high (90%-95%) long-term patency. In selected patients, angioplasty and/or stent placement can be performed with an expectation of good short-term and mid-term results. This particular lesion, with adherent thrombus that could potentially embolize to the vertebrobasilar circulation or to the distal upper-extremity vessels, would be a fairly poor candidate lesion for endovascular management.

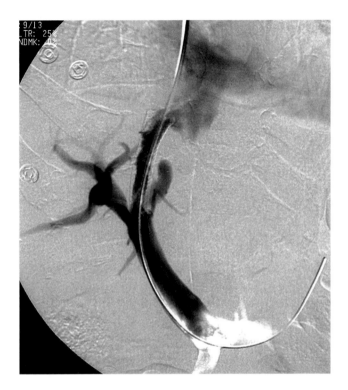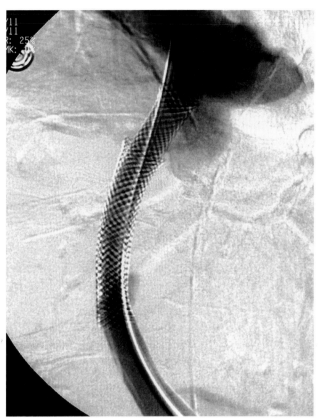

1. What interventional procedure was previously performed in this patient?

2. Name two common indications for this procedure.

3. Name two important early complications of this procedure.

4. What common cause of late failure of this therapy is depicted in the first image?

Post-TIPS Stenosis

1. Transjugular intrahepatic portosystemic shunt (TIPS) placement.

2. Variceal hemorrhage and refractory ascites.

3. Intraperitoneal hemorrhage, development or progression of hepatic encephalopathy.

4. Stenosis at the hepatic vein end of the stent and within the stent.

Reference

Patel NH. Portal hypertension. *Semin Roentgenol.* 2002; 37(4):293-302.

Cross-Reference

Vascular and Interventional Radiology: THE REQUISITES, pp 391-399.

Comment

TIPS is commonly performed in patients with portal hypertension and recurrent variceal bleeding after failed endoscopic therapy, refractory ascites, and/or hepatic hydrothorax. To perform TIPS, a catheter is placed in a hepatic vein (usually the right) via an internal jugular vein approach. A directional needle is passed through the hepatic parenchyma into the portal venous system (usually the right portal vein). Following portal venography and pressure measurements, the hepatic tract is angioplastied, and a stent is placed bridging the hepatic tract from the portal vein to the hepatic vein.

Major early complications of TIPS include intraperitoneal hemorrhage due to transcapsular needle puncture, worsening of hepatic encephalopathy due to shunting of blood away from the liver via the TIPS, stent infection with sepsis (rare), and early TIPS occlusion. For these reasons, relative contraindications to TIPS include pre-existing hepatic encephalopathy, hepatic failure, uncorrected coagulopathy, and active infection.

Early TIPS occlusion is often caused by a fistulous connection with the biliary tree; this can now be treated with placement of a stent graft to exclude the biliary–TIPS fistula.

The 1-year patency rate for TIPS is about 50%. The most common cause of long-term TIPS failure is the development of stenosis along the course of the TIPS, most commonly at the hepatic vein end but also at the portal vein end or within the stent. When this occurs, variceal bleeding or ascites can recur. For this reason, post-TIPS duplex ultrasound surveillance is performed at regular intervals in order to identify developing stenoses. When abnormally low or high flow velocities are present within or adjacent to the TIPS, the patient is referred for TIPS venography. TIPS stenoses or occlusions can be effectively treated with balloon angioplasty or repeat stent placement.

Notes

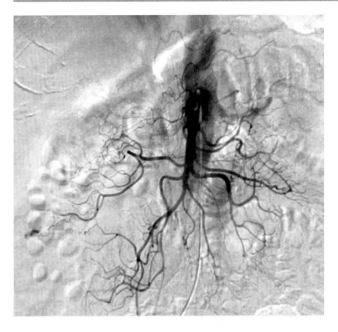 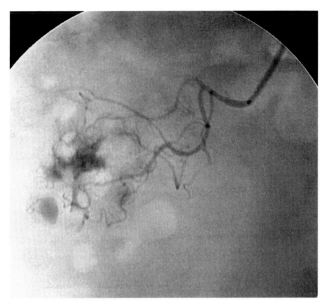

1. What arteriographic abnormality is present?

2. What is the endovascular treatment of choice?

3. If superselective catheterization is not successful, what endovascular pharmacologic therapy could be recommended?

4. What are the contraindications to this form of therapy?

Lower Gastrointestinal (Diverticular) Bleed

1. Active extravasation from a branch of the right colic artery.

2. Coil embolization of the bleeding branch.

3. Vasopressin infusion.

4. Severe coronary artery disease, dysrhythmia, cerebrovascular disease, severe hypertension.

Reference

Darcy M. Treatment of lower gastrointestinal (LGI) bleeding: Vasopressin infusion versus embolization. *J Vasc Intervent Radiol.* 2003;14:535-543.

Cross-Reference

Vascular and Interventional Radiology: THE REQUISITES, pp 298-304.

Comment

Catheter-directed vasopressin infusion has traditionally been the first-line treatment for LGI bleeding. This is based on findings in older literature in which infarction often complicated LGI embolization. With modern embolization techniques, clinically significant bowel ischemia has become an uncommon complication. Although the efficacies of vasopressin and embolization are fairly comparable, embolotherapy has advantages in terms of quicker completion of therapy and decreased likelihood of systemic complications. Although vasopressin is still probably preferable for diffuse lesions and cases in which superselective catheterization is not technically possible, embolization should be considered a primary option for treating LGI bleeding.

Vasopressin is a natural hormone that reduces pulse pressure and blood flow via constriction of smooth muscle in splanchnic blood vessels and bowel wall, allowing clot to form.

After a bleeding site is identified, a catheter is secured with its tip in a central vessel supplying the bleeding site; in this case, the tip would be located in the proximal superior mesenteric artery. Vasopressin infusion is started at 0.2 U/min. Follow-up arteriography is performed in 20 to 30 minutes to assess response. If active extravasation is still present, the infusion is increased to 0.4 U/min, and arteriography is again repeated in 20 to 30 minutes. If active extravasation is still observed, alternative therapies (such as embolization) should be pursued. If vasopressin infusion does result in cessation of bleeding, the infusion is continued for 12 to 24 hours and the patient is closely monitored in an intensive care unit. Mild abdominal discomfort at the initiation of infusion is common, but persistent pain might indicate ischemia, signaling the need to reduce the infusion rate. If continued cessation of bleeding is observed clinically, then the vasopressin infusion is tapered over the next 12 to 24 hours.

Initial success rates for vasopressin infusion therapy in controlling LGI bleeding range from 60% to 90%, but rebleeding occurs in approximately 40%. Vasopressin is not effective in the treatment of upper gastrointestinal bleeding, and it is rarely used in that setting.

Notes

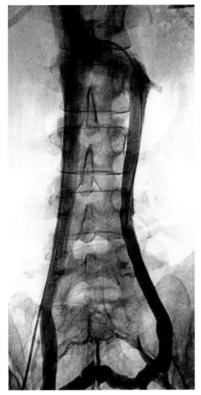

Courtesy of Dr. Thomas Vesely.

1. What anatomic variant is present?

2. How common is this anomaly?

3. Why is this significant during placement of an inferior vena cava (IVC) filter?

4. What potential solutions exist?

Variant Anatomy: Duplicated Inferior Vena Cava

1. Duplicated IVC.

2. Approximately 2%.

3. Failure to recognize the vascular duplication and insertion of an infrarenal IVC filter into the right-sided cava alone can permit pulmonary embolism from a left lower extremity thrombus.

4. Either place one filter in each IVC (two filters total) or place a suprarenal filter.

Reference

Hicks ME, Malden ES, Vesely TM, et al Prospective anatomic study of the inferior vena cava and renal veins: Comparison of selective renal venography with cavography and relevance in filter placement. *J Vasc Intervent Radiol*. 1995;6:721-729.

Cross-Reference

Vascular and Interventional Radiology: THE REQUI-SITES, pp 350-355.

Comment

Normally a single IVC drains the lower extremities and iliac veins. However, several congenital anomalies of venous development exist and can affect IVC filter placement. Therefore, an inferior vena cavogram should always be performed before deploying a filter.

In patients with duplication of the IVC, the left-sided IVC accepts drainage from the left renal and adrenal veins and subsequently drains into the right-sided IVC at the L1-L2 level. Therefore, to achieve adequate protection against potential pulmonary emboli originating in both limbs, it is necessary either to place two filters (one in each IVC) or to place a single (suprarenal) filter above the confluence of the two IVCs.

A solitary left-sided IVC is less common, occurring in 0.2% of persons. Similar to the duplicated IVC, this vessel drains to the right at the level of the renal veins.

Congenital absence of the IVC is seen in 0.6% of patients with congenital heart disease but is more common with cyanotic heart disease. Typically, the hepatic segment of the IVC is interrupted and lower-extremity venous drainage occurs via the azygous and hemiazygous systems. The hepatic veins drain directly to the right atrium.

Notes

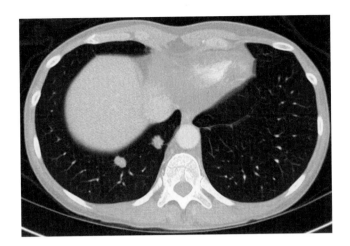

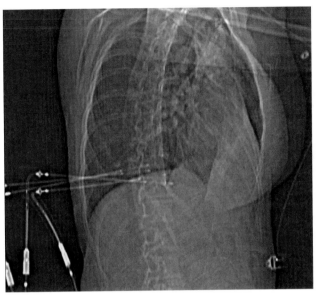

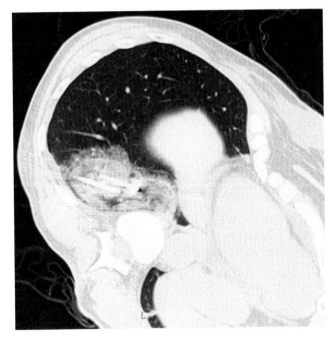

1. What is the diagnosis in this patient with a history of colon cancer?

2. What procedure is being performed in the second and third images?

3. What potential complications are associated with this procedure?

4. What other local therapies can be used to treat these lesions?

Lung Metastases: Cryoablation

1. Metastatic lung nodules.

2. Cryoablation.

3. Hemoptysis, pneumothorax, hemothorax.

4. Wedge resection, radiofrequency ablation, and external beam radiation.

References

Wang H, Littrup PJ, Duan Y, et al. Thoracic masses treated with percutaneous cryotherapy: Initial experience with more than 200 procedures. *Radiology*. 2005;235:289-298.

Kawamura M, Izumi Y, Tsukada N, et al. Percutaneous cryoablation of small pulmonary malignant tumors under computed tomographic guidance with local anesthesia for nonsurgical candidates. *J Thorac Cardiovasc Surg*. 2006;131:1007-1013.

Goldberg SN, Charboneau JW, Dodd 3rd GD, et al. International Working Group on Image-Guided Tumor Ablation: Image-guided tumor ablation: Proposal for standardization of terms and reporting criteria. *Radiology*. 2003;228:335-345.

Comment

The standard of care for metastatic lung nodules with no extrapulmonary involvement is surgical resection: wedge resection, lobectomy, or even pneumonectomy. Many patients with metastatic lung disease are not candidates for surgery owing to poor pulmonary reserve or general health condition. Less-invasive therapies such as cryoablation, radiofrequency ablation, or external beam radiation can be offered to these patients. Local ablative therapies have a further advantage over external beam radiation in that they can be repeated as needed for lesions that develop further along in the course of the disease, as is typically seen in patients with metastatic disease.

Cryoablation involves freezing and rapid thawing of tissue that leads to cell membrane disruption, resulting in cell death. The application of cryoablation includes tumors in many locations including lung, kidney, liver, bone, soft tissues, and others. Image guidance with CT or US is used for placement of the cryoprobes, and the freezing and thawing is monitored by CT imaging. Lung consolidation is clearly seen in the area exposed to freezing in the third image.

Hemoptysis occurs commonly; however, this is minimal in the majority of patients and requires no further intervention aside from patient reassurance. Owing to the relatively large size of the cryoprobes, pneumothorax is a common procedural complication, with rates reported at 50% to 62%. Chest tube placement is only needed in 12% of these patients.

Notes

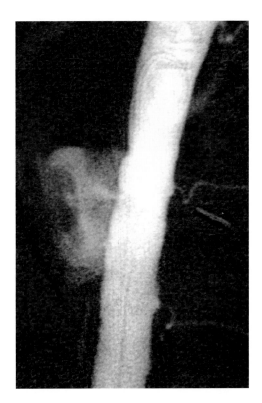 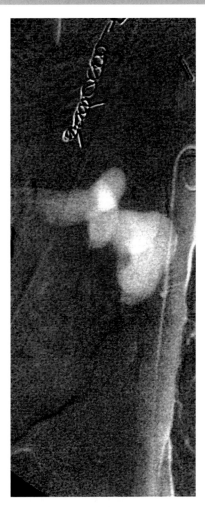

1. What is the diagnosis in this patient with recurrent gastrointestinal (GI) bleeding?

2. What procedure did this patient likely undergo in the past?

3. What structure is opacified in the second image?

4. How are these patients usually treated?

Aortoenteric Fistula

1. Aortoenteric fistula.

2. An aortic vascular procedure, such as repair of an abdominal aortic aneurysm.

3. Duodenum.

4. Graft removal with closure of the aortic stump, repair of the bowel defect, interposition of viable tissue (e.g., omentum) between the aorta and the bowel, and extraanatomic bypass grafting for lower-extremity revascularization.

Reference

Lemos JD Raffetto TC, et al. Primary aortoduodenal fistula: A case report and review of the literature. *J Vasc Surg.* 2003;37:686-689.

Cross-Reference

Vascular and Interventional Radiology: THE REQUISITES, pp 252-261.

Comment

Formation of an aortoenteric fistula is much more common as an infrequent (0.4%-2.4%) complication of aortic vascular procedures (termed *secondary*) than as a complication of aneurysm rupture (termed *primary*). In either situation, this disorder carries a significant risk of death or limb loss despite treatment. Patients with a direct communication between the anastomotic suture line of the aortic graft and the adjacent bowel lumen (graft–enteric fistula) often present with intermittent hematemesis or melena days to weeks after the procedure. Patients with an erosion remote from the suture line with exposure of a portion of the graft prosthesis (graft–enteric erosion) commonly present with chronic GI bleeding. Patients with lesser degrees of bleeding can present with septicemia resulting from graft infection.

Most cases occur two or more years after the aortic surgery. For this reason, although aortography is not routinely performed in the angiographic evaluation of all GI bleeding patients, those with a suitable history should be studied with aortography. Most cases involve the third or fourth portions of the duodenum (as in this case) owing to the proximity of the graft anastomosis to this fairly fixated portion of bowel, but in 10% to 20% the more distal small bowel or colon is involved. Endoscopy is the preferred first step in evaluation because it can diagnose many other more-common causes of GI bleeding, and rarely it can provide a definitive diagnosis by visualizing a focus of exposed graft.

Notes

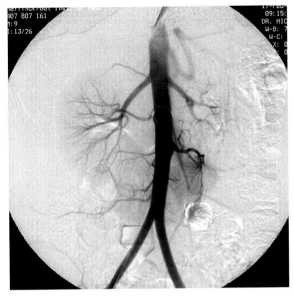

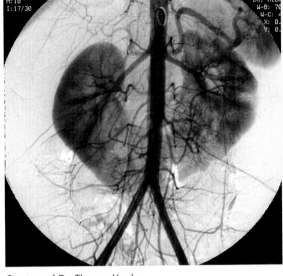

Courtesy of Dr. Thomas Vesely.

Courtesy of Dr. Thomas Vesely.

1. What congenital variant is present?

2. How common is this variant?

3. Is the renal arterial anatomy usually normal?

4. Is this more common in men or women?

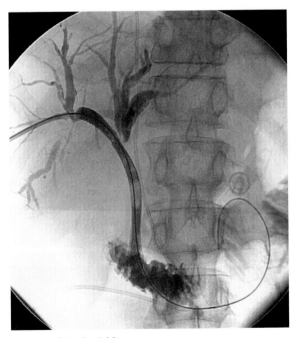

Courtesy of Dr. Daniel Brown.

1. What device has been inserted?

2. Is this a temporary or permanent device?

3. Is this device typically used for benign or malignant disorders?

4. In the case above, will the entire biliary ductal system be adequately drained?

CASE 73

Horseshoe Kidney

1. Horseshoe kidney.

2. 1 in 500 to 700 autopsies.

3. Usually not.

4. More common in men (2:1 ratio).

References

Raj GV, Auge BK, Weizer AZ. Percutaneous management of calculi within horseshoe kidneys. *J Urol.* 2003;170:48-51.

Cross-Reference

Vascular and Interventional Radiology: THE REQUISITES, pp 323-325.

Comment

In a horseshoe kidney, the two kidneys are joined at either the lower pole (90%) or upper pole (10%) by a parenchymal–fibrous isthmus. Typically, the long axis of each kidney is oriented somewhat more medially than normal, and the renal pelves and ureters exit their respective kidneys anteriorly. The vascular supply is often aberrant and often there are multiple renal arteries (six or more renal arteries are possible). In the case presented here, at least three renal arteries supply the right kidney, one left renal artery is present, and one more artery can be seen to supply at least part of the isthmus that joins the lower poles of the kidneys.

A primary complication of horseshoe kidney is the development of renal calculi. Other associations include genitourinary abnormalities such as caudal ectopia, vesicoureteral reflux, hydronephrosis, ureteral duplication, hypospadias, undescended testis, and anomalies of the cardiovascular, skeletal, central nervous, and gastrointestinal systems.

CASE 74

Metallic Biliary Stent Placement

1. Wallstent.

2. Permanent.

3. Malignant.

4. Probably not, but unilateral drainage will probably be sufficient to palliate obstructive symptoms.

Reference

Schmassmann A, Von Gunten E, Knuchel J, et al. Wallstents versus plastic stents in malignant biliary obstruction: Effects of stent patency of the first and second stent upon patient compliance and survival. *Am J Gastroenterol.* 1996;91:654-659.

Cross-Reference

Vascular and Interventional Radiology: THE REQUISITES, pp 561-577.

Comment

There are a wide variety of causes of biliary ductal obstruction or stricture. Benign causes include operative trauma, biliary ductal stones, scarring from prior passage of biliary stones, chronic pancreatitis, external compression, and nonoperative trauma. Malignant causes include cholangiocarcinoma, gallbladder cancer, pancreatic head carcinoma, ampullary neoplasms, and metastatic porta hepatis lymphadenopathy.

Completely internalized biliary stents are often preferred to external or internal–external drainage catheters. However, because of the viscous nature of biliary secretions, all biliary stents must be changed regularly to prevent occlusion of the stent and/or formation of calculi. For this reason, the vast majority of internal stents and all stents placed for benign causes are made of catheter-type materials such as silicone rubber (Silastic). Permanent metallic stents should only be inserted for palliation of malignant obstructions in patients with short anticipated life expectancy.

The imaging in this case demonstrates extension of a metallic stent from the right main hepatic duct into the duodenum. A focal narrowing and obstruction persists at the distal left main bile duct, with contrast stasis in the left bile ducts from the cholangiogram. Fortunately, it is not necessary to drain the entire biliary ductal system to obtain symptom relief from pain, jaundice, and pruritus, so the obstructed left ducts can be left undrained unless infection later occurs in the left system.

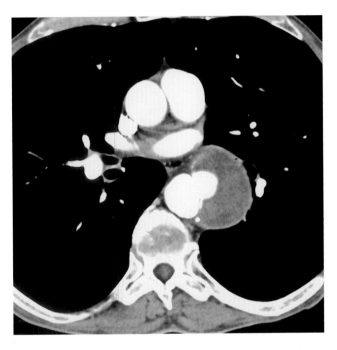 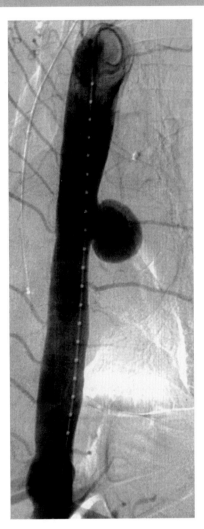

1. What is the diagnosis?

2. Where does this problem occur most often?

3. Name two major complications of this problem.

4. Why was the angiogram obtained?

Penetrating Aortic Ulcer

1. Penetrating ulcer of the thoracic aorta.

2. Descending thoracic aorta.

3. Dissection and rupture.

4. To plan endovascular therapy.

Reference

Ganaha F, Miller DC, Sugimoto K, et al. Prognosis of aortic intramural hematoma with and without penetrating atherosclerotic ulcer: A clinical and radiological analysis. *Circulation*. 2002;106(3):342-348.

Cross-Reference

Vascular and Interventional Radiology: THE REQUISITES, pp 231-233.

Comment

The first image demonstrates a focal outpouching of contrast from the thoracic aorta with an associated pseudoaneurysm. The second image confirms the presence of a focal contrast collection with a narrow neck that protrudes from the descending thoracic aorta. The findings in this patient, who presented with acute chest pain, are consistent with a penetrating atherosclerotic aortic ulcer.

Penetrating atherosclerotic ulcer represents one entity within a spectrum of aortic disorders, which also encompasses aortic intramural hematoma and aortic dissection. A significant percentage of patients with symptomatic penetrating atherosclerotic ulcer do progress to aortic dissection, and some patients progress to aortic rupture. The presence of left-sided hemothorax on a CT scan is therefore of significant concern.

The conventional treatment for this disorder is surgical aortic repair. However, thoracotomy and descending thoracic aortic repair are associated with considerable risk of death, paraplegia, and other major morbidities. For this reason, selected patients with this disease are now treated with placement of an endovascular stent graft. The patient depicted here would be an excellent candidate for this procedure, because the aorta is straight and not excessively enlarged, the ulcer defect is short, and the surrounding aorta appears reasonably free of bulky atherosclerotic plaque.

Notes

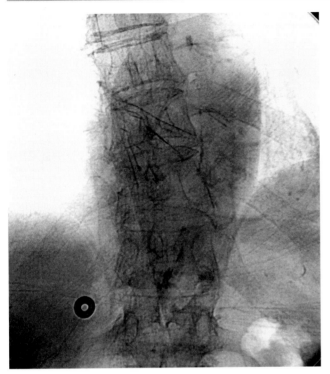

Courtesy of Dr. James Duncan.

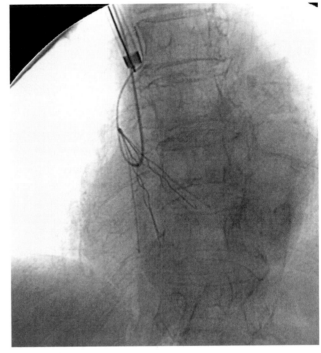

Courtesy of Dr. James Duncan.

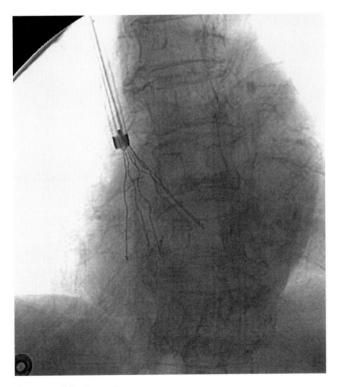

Courtesy of Dr. James Duncan.

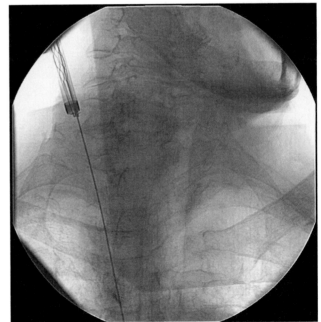

Courtesy of Dr. James Duncan.

1. What abnormality is depicted in the first image?

2. Is this likely to become symptomatic?

3. What do you recommend?

4. What device is most commonly used for this procedure?

Foreign Body Retrieval

1. Foreign body (a Greenfield inferor vena cava [IVC] filter) within the right atrium.

2. Yes.

3. Transcatheter retrieval.

4. Amplatz nitinol gooseneck snare (Microvena, White Bear Lake, Minn).

Reference
Gabelmann A, Kramer S, Gorich J. Percutaneous retrieval of lost or misplaced intravascular objects. *Am J Roentgenol.* 2001;176:1509-1513.

Cross-Reference
Vascular and Interventional Radiology: THE REQUISITES, pp 114-116.

Comment
A variety of intravascular foreign bodies have been described, including catheter and guidewire fragments, filters, stents, coils, and balloon and bullet fragments. Objects lodge in a location corresponding to their size, flexibility, and shape. Intravenous objects commonly lodge within the superior vena cava, right heart, or pulmonary artery.

Large intravascular foreign bodies (as in this case) and small foreign bodies that have been present for a short time are typically removed to eliminate the potential complications of arrhythmia, thrombosis, bacteremia, and vascular or cardiac perforation. Small objects that have been present for prolonged periods can become incorporated into the vessel wall or endocardium, and they are often left alone unless they are causing complications.

Transcatheter retrieval is the preferred treatment. The site of percutaneous entry is selected based upon the location and orientation of the foreign body. A sheath should be inserted to minimize trauma to the access vessel when the object is removed. Typically, a guiding catheter and snare device are used. Preferably, the foreign body is snared near its tip, the snare loop is snugged around the fragment, and the object is withdrawn into the sheath and out of the vessel in a single motion. On occasion, a cutdown may be necessary to remove large objects or objects with sharp edges.

Notes

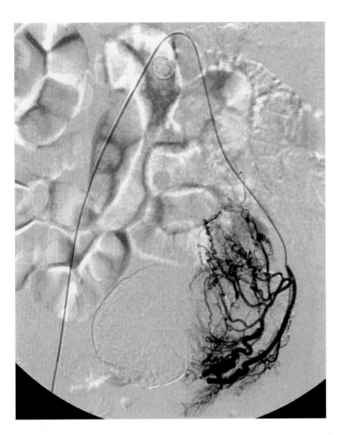

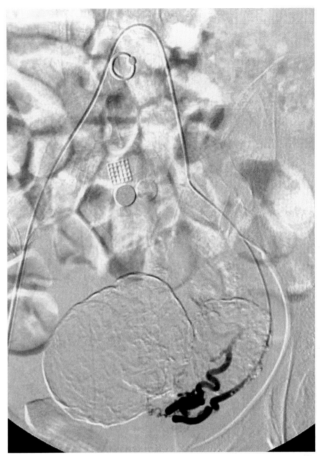

1. What vessel has been selected for the angiogram in the first image?

2. From what parent artery does this vessel arise?

3. What symptoms is this patient likely experiencing?

4. Why is arteriography being performed?

Uterine Fibroid Embolization

1. Left uterine artery.

2. Anterior division of the left internal iliac artery.

3. Menorrhagia, pelvic pain or discomfort, and/or urinary frequency.

4. To facilitate uterine artery embolization.

Reference
Pron G, Bennett J, Common A, et al. The Ontario Uterine Fibroid Embolization Trial. Part 2. Uterine fibroid reduction and symptom relief after uterine artery embolization for fibroids. *Fertil Steril*. 2003;79:120-127.

Cross-Reference
Vascular and Interventional Radiology: THE REQUISITES, pp 280-282.

Comment
Uterine arteriography and embolization therapy can be performed for a variety of indications: (1) To control postpartum bleeding refractory to medical management; (2) To control postoperative bleeding after cesarean section or other procedures; (3) To treat trauma-related pelvic hemorrhage; (4) To improve symptoms in women with uterine fibroids (uterine fibroid embolization, or UFE); (5) To palliate bleeding pelvic malignancies (although bleeding commonly recurs in this situation).

Uterine fibroid tumors occur in 20% to 40% of women older than 35 years, but they cause significant symptoms only in a minority of patients. The symptoms are usually initially treated with hormonal agents, but long-term use of these agents can be associated with unfavorable side effects. Hysterectomy has long been the mainstay of therapy, but in recent years myomectomy (removal of one or more fibroids) has been used in patients desiring to preserve the uterus. Myomectomy, however, is associated with a fairly high incidence of bleeding complications when performed for multiple fibroids, and a high recurrence rate has been observed.

For this reason, UFE has evolved into an excellent alternative therapy for women with symptomatic uterine fibroids who desire to preserve the uterus. UFE is associated with 85% to 90% success in producing significant improvement in symptoms of menorrhagia and/or pelvic pain, and it has been associated with improvements in health-related quality of life. Compared with hysterectomy, UFE is associated with less blood loss, decreased hospital stay, and decreased major complications.

Notes

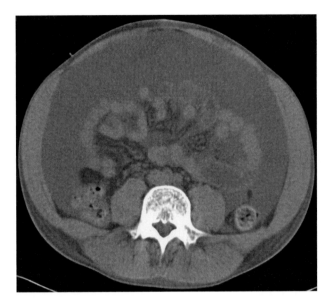

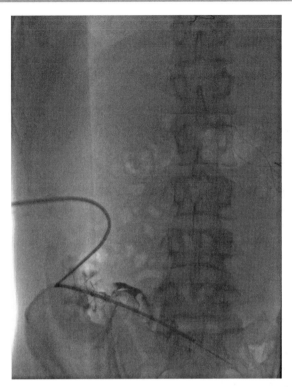

1. What is the primary abnormality seen on the first image?

2. What symptoms is this patient likely experiencing?

3. What procedure was performed in the second image?

4. What is the potential long-term complication of this procedure?

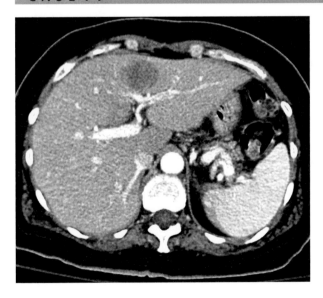

1. Describe the abnormality.

2. What is the differential diagnosis?

3. How is the definitive diagnosis of this lesion made?

4. What imaging modalities could be used to assist image-guided biopsy?

CASE 78

Massive Ascites: Tunneled Peritoneal Catheter Placement

1. Massive ascites.

2. Abdominal distention, dyspnea, and fatigue.

3. Tunneled peritoneal catheter placement.

4. Bacterial peritonitis.

Reference

O'NeillMJ, Weissleder R, Gervais DA, et al. Tunneled peritoneal catheter placement under sonographic and fluoroscopic guidance in the palliative treatment of malignant ascites. *AJR Am J Roentgenol.* 2001; 177:615-618.

Comment

Massive ascites can develop secondary to a variety of etiologies including portal hypertension, malignant ascites, and right-sided heart failure (as in this case). The accumulation of fluid in the peritoneal cavity causes abdominal distention, which in extreme cases can result in increased pressure on the diaphragm, leading to dyspnea and easy fatigability. This can greatly affect the patient's quality of life.

Medical management with diuretics is the first-line treatment. Patients might also require therapeutic paracentesis to remove the accumulated ascites. In patients who fail to get relief of their symptoms from these measures, those who require frequent large-volume paracentesis, and those who suffer adverse effects of diuretic therapy (impaired renal function), other therapies are indicated. Transjugular intrahepatic portosystemic shunt (TIPS) can be performed for patients with portal hypertension; however, for patients with malignant ascites or ascites secondary to severe right-sided heart failure, placement of a tunneled peritoneal catheter is the procedure of choice.

The procedure is performed similar to tunneled central venous catheter placement with the exception that the catheter is placed within the peritoneal cavity and tunneled through the soft tissues of the anterior abdominal wall. The patient can then easily drain the ascitic fluid by opening the clamp intermittently as needed. Bacterial peritonitis is a rare but serious potential complication.

CASE 79

Percutaneous Transabdominal Liver Biopsy (Focal Lesion)

1. Hypoattenuating lesion in the left liver lobe, likely a solid mass.

2. Hepatocellular carcinoma, focal nodular hyperplasia, hepatic adenoma, metastasis.

3. Biopsy.

4. Ultrasound, CT, MRI.

Reference

Shankar S, Van Sonnenberg E, Silverman SG, et al. Interventional radiology procedures in the liver. Biopsy, drainage, and ablation. *Clin Liver Dis.* 2002;6:91-118.

Cross-Reference

Vascular and Interventional Radiology: THE REQUISITES, pp 469-476.

Comment

Noninvasive imaging of solid hepatic lesions is often unable to exclude the possibility of primary or metastatic malignant disease. For this reason, tissue biopsy is often indicated. For focal liver lesions, biopsy is performed from a percutaneous transabdominal route. Fine-needle aspiration and core biopsy specimens may be obtained.

The potential complications of liver biopsy include severe intraperitoneal hemorrhage, hemobilia, and pneumothorax. Accordingly, preprocedure precautions should ensure that coagulation parameters and platelet level are within normal limits, particularly in patients with hepatic cirrhosis. In addition, for lesions located high within the liver parenchyma, the route of access should be carefully planned to avoid traversing the lateral sulcus of the right pleural space. For left-sided lesions, the proximity of the pericardium should be similarly kept in mind.

Ultrasound or CT are used for the vast majority of image-guided biopsies. Ultrasound provides the advantage of real-time needle visualization and is less costly than using CT. On the other hand, many lesions are not clearly visible on ultrasound, making CT a better choice in these cases. MRI guidance is being used in some centers, primarily for hepatic dome lesions in which its multiplanar capability can be advantageous.

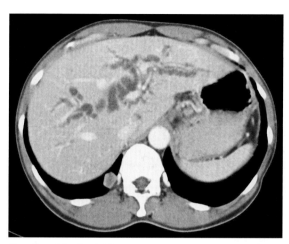

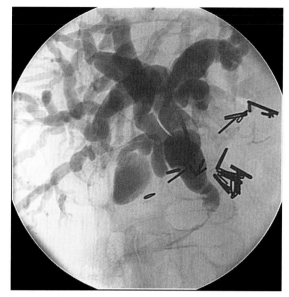

Courtesy of Dr. Daniel Brown.

Courtesy of Dr. Daniel Brown.

1. What is the probable underlying diagnosis causing biliary obstruction?

2. What symptoms does this patient most likely have?

3. How might the interventionalist contribute to obtaining a definitive diagnosis?

4. Are bilateral drainage catheters needed?

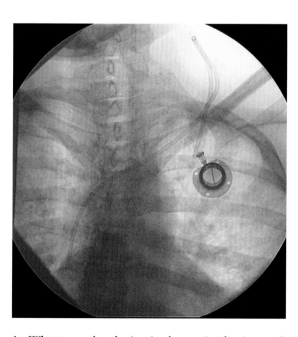

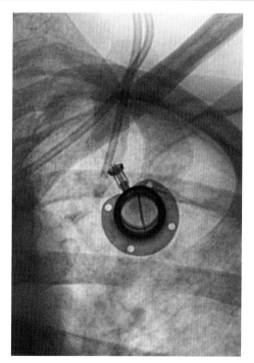

1. What vascular device is shown in the images?

2. What problem is identified and how did this occur?

3. Name two other mechanical problems of these devices.

4. For what type of patient is this device typically used?

CASE 80

Malignant Common Bile Duct Stricture

1. Pancreatic head adenocarcinoma or cholangiocarcinoma.

2. Painless jaundice, weight loss.

3. Biliary brush biopsy.

4. No. The right and left biliary systems communicate in this case, so only one catheter is needed.

Reference

Govil H, Reddy V, Kluskens L, et al. Brush cytology of the biliary tract: Retrospective study of 278 cases with histopathologic correlation. *Diagn Cytopathol.* 2002; 26(5):273-277.

Cross-Reference

Vascular and Interventional Radiology: THE REQUISITES, pp 561-577.

Comment

Malignant biliary obstruction may be produced by pancreatic carcinoma, cholangiocarcinoma, gallbladder cancer, intrahepatic metastatic disease, or portal hepatic nodal disease causing extrinsic common bile duct (CBD) compression. Although the clinical context must always be taken into account, the irregular rat-tail appearance of this distal CBD stricture is highly suggestive of a malignant etiology.

The interventional radiologist might have several tasks to complete in managing the patient with malignant CBD obstruction: (1) Percutaneous transhepatic cholangiography can outline the extent of the biliary abnormality and allow selection of a duct to use for definitive biliary access; (2) Biliary drainage can be performed to treat cholangitis, prevent episodes of biliary sepsis, and relieve obstructive symptoms including jaundice and pruritus; (3) Although its diagnostic sensitivity for pancreatic or biliary adenocarcinoma is only 50% to 70%, biliary brush biopsy can sometimes provide a definitive tissue diagnosis; (4) If the malignancy is unresectable and the patient has short life expectancy, a metallic (permanent) stent can be placed to facilitate internal drainage and thereby allow removal of the externally protruding biliary drainage catheter(s).

CASE 81

Port Separation

1. Implantable port catheter.

2. Separation of the two components of an attachable-type port.

3. Flipping of the port within its pocket, kinking, proximal migration.

4. Patients in need of long-term, intermittent access.

Reference

Funaki B, Szymski GX, Hackworth CA, et al. Radiologic placement of subcutaneous infusion chest ports for long-term central venous access. *Am J Roentgenol.* 1997;169:1431-1434.

Cross-Reference

Vascular and Interventional Radiology: THE REQUISITES, pp 174-181.

Comment

In addition to the general complications of central venous access described earlier, a variety of device-specific complications can occur. This case demonstrates one device-specific complication of a port catheter: separation of the port and catheter components of the device. In addition, this particular catheter has been placed with an unfavorable upward curve, which may be partly extravascular.

Several types of port catheter devices are available. In many institutions, single-piece devices are used, and in other institutions, double-piece or attachable ports are used. The attachable ports are typically assembled by the physician when the port is placed. In occasional instances, presumably related to poor initial technique in attaching the pieces and/or to local trauma, the two components can separate. This is important, because any fluid injected into the port will extravasate into the chest wall. The separation can be fixed by reopening the port incision, dissecting down to the port and catheter, and reattaching the components. Alternatively, the port can be replaced with a completely new device.

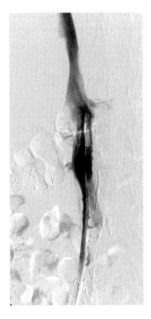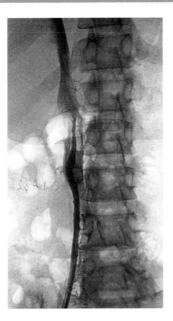

1. What problem is identified on injection of this hemodialysis catheter?

2. Which is more likely to be present: problems with aspiration or with injection?

3. Is catheter exchange over a guidewire likely to result in long-term improvement?

4. Why was this long-term dialysis catheter placed from the common femoral vein?

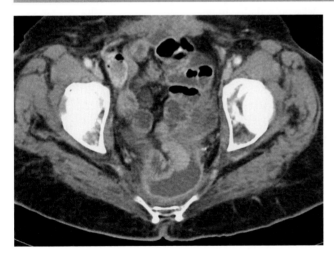

1. What treatment options are available for the abnormality shown?

2. What routes of access can be used to drain a pelvic fluid collection?

3. For each of these routes of access, what imaging modalities are typically used to facilitate drainage?

4. Name two potential undesirable sequelae of transgluteal abscess drainage.

CASE 82

Pericatheter Fibrin Sheath

1. Fibrin sheath.

2. Aspiration.

3. No.

4. The internal jugular veins are probably occluded.

Reference

Gray RJ, Levitin A, Buck D, et al. Percutaneous fibrin sheath stripping versus transcatheter urokinase infusion for malfunctioning well-positioned tunneled central venous dialysis catheters: A prospective, randomized trial. *J Vasc Interv Radiol.* 2000;11:1121-1129.

Cross-Reference

Vascular and Interventional Radiology: THE REQUISITES, pp 174-181.

Comment

Central venous catheters are prone to problems including infection, end-hole occlusion, venous thrombosis, malposition, migration, kinking, vessel wall damage, and catheter fracture. One of the most common and difficult problems is the development of a fibrin sheath around the catheter tip. Shortly after placement, virtually all catheters become covered by a layer of fibrin, which eventually forms a sleeve around the catheter. When this obstructs the catheter end hole and/or side holes, the usual clinical finding is impaired ability to aspirate blood but preserved ability to inject. Dialysis catheters often demonstrate diminished flow rates in this situation. The typical venographic appearance is observed in this case: Contrast flows retrograde along the catheter within the fibrin sheath, outlining the catheter.

Treatment options vary. Catheter exchange over a guidewire can be performed, but it is unlikely to produce long-term improvement because the catheter is typically reinserted into the existing fibrin sheath. Alternatively, low-dose thrombolytic agents can be used, either via instillation in the catheter for 30 to 60 minutes or via infusion for several hours. Some advocate disrupting the fibrin sheath using guidewire or angioplasty balloon manipulation or stripping the fibrin sheath using a snare device inserted from another access vein. Unfortunately, most treatments lead to only temporary relief because the fibrin sheath tends to re-form over time.

CASE 83

Percutaneous Drainage of Deep Pelvic Abscess

1. Surgical abscess drainage or percutaneous image-guided abscess drainage.

2. Transabdominal, transgluteal, transvaginal, transrectal, and transperineal.

3. Transvaginal, transrectal, and transperineal drainage are generally performed under combination US/fluoroscopic guidance. Transabdominal and transgluteal abscess drainage can be performed under CT or ultrasound/fluoroscopy. CT is commonly used for transgluteal drainage.

4. Pelvic arterial hemorrhage, pain.

Reference

Hovsepian DM. Transrectal and transvaginal abscess drainage. *J Vasc Intervent Radiol.* 1997;8:501-515.

Cross-Reference

Vascular and Interventional Radiology: THE REQUISITES, pp 506-508.

Comment

The first-line management of deep pelvic abscesses is usually percutaneous imaging-guided drainage. Because of the presence of small bowel, bladder, and other structures within the pelvis, a simple transabdominal access route is often not available.

In choosing a potential access route, the first question to ask is whether a draining sinus is present. If so, then the abscess cavity may be defined by contrast injection directly into the skin defect; in this situation a catheter can usually be advanced under fluoroscopy into the abscess without the need for needle puncture. When this option does not exist, careful examination of the CT scan is critical in planning therapy.

When a direct transabdominal route into the collection is not present, the transvaginal and transrectal access routes are usually considered next in the absence of contraindications (e.g., a surgical bowel anastomosis in the rectal area). The advantages of the transvaginal and transrectal routes are their usual close proximity to the fluid collection and the lower risk of complications (bleeding and pain) compared with transgluteal drainage. Additionally, transgluteal drainage is occasionally technically difficult when the collection is small, because the window into the collection must be crossed with pinpoint accuracy to avoid traversing surrounding bowel and pelvic organs.

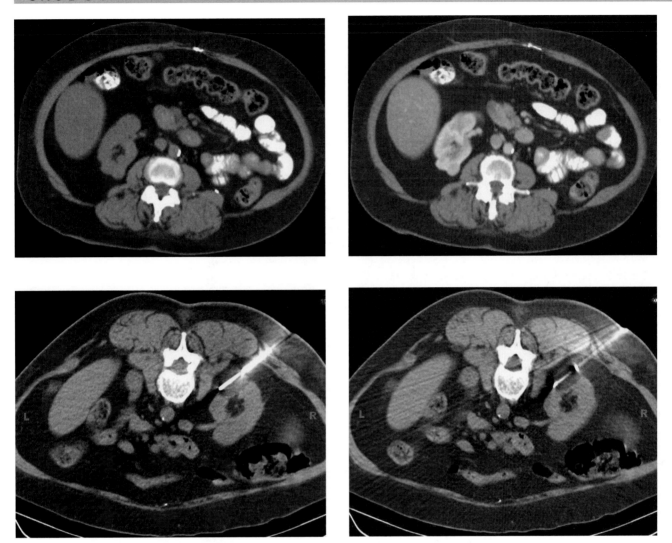

1. What abnormalities are present on the first two images?

2. What is the most likely diagnosis?

3. What treatment options are available for this patient?

4. What procedure is being performed in the last image?

Renal Cell Carcinoma: Percutaneous Cryoablation

1. Solid enhancing partially exophytic mass arising from the superior pole of the right kidney and nonvisualization of the left kidney with the presence of a surgical clip in the left retroperitoneum.

2. This patient previously underwent a radical left nephrectomy for renal cell carcinoma.
A contralateral enhancing solid renal mass is identified consistent with renal cell carcinoma.

3. Nephron-sparing therapies include partial nephrectomy (open or laparoscopic), laparoscopic cryoablation, and percutaneous cryoablation or radiofrequency ablation.

4. Percutaneous cryoablation.

Reference

Atwell TD, Farrell MA, Callstrom MR, et al. Percutaneous cryoablation of large renal masses: Technical feasibility and short-term outcome. *AJR Am J Roentgenol.* 2007;188:1195-2000.

Comment

Renal tumors are being found incidentally at an increasing rate. This has allowed detection of these tumors at earlier stages where tumors are much smaller. Surgical resection of these tumors remains the standard of care. This comprises radical and partial nephrectomy, which may be performed in an open manner or laparoscopically.

Nephron-sparing therapies have gained favor in recent years for preservation of renal function. These treatments include partial nephrectomy, laparoscopic cryoablation, and percutaneous image-guided cryoablation and radiofrequency ablation. Percutaneous ablations have obvious advantages over open or laparoscopic surgical procedures including decreased morbidity and the potential for being performed under moderate sedation.

Percutaneous cryoablation was the chosen therapy for the patient in this case to treat the tumor in her solitary kidney for its nephron-sparing potential and the lack of need for general anesthesia because she had many comorbid conditions, placing her at increased risk for morbidity from a surgical procedure. Ultrasound or CT guidance can be used for placement of the cryoprobes, and the freezing and thawing of the tumor is monitored with CT surveillance, which clearly demonstrates the formation of the ice ball around the cryoprobe (low-attenuation area seen in the fourth image).

Notes

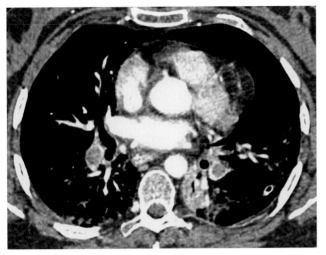

Courtesy of Dr. James Duncan.

1. What abnormality is present on this chest CT scan?

2. Is this problem likely acute or chronic?

3. What are the potential advantages of CT in evaluating this clinical problem?

4. What is the primary pitfall of CT in evaluating this clinical problem?

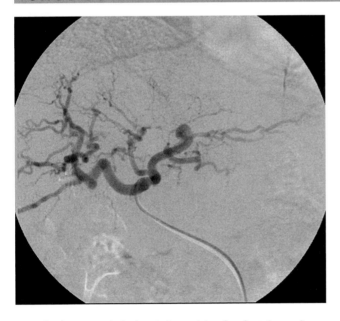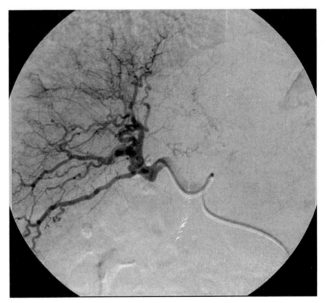

1. Which artery is being injected in the first image?

2. How is this arteriogram abnormal?

3. What diagnosis is likely?

4. Is flow through this vessel increased or decreased in this condition?

CASE 85

Acute Pulmonary Embolism on CT Angiography

1. Bilateral pulmonary embolism (PE).

2. Acute.

3. CT is noninvasive compared with angiography, it provides more direct visualization of thrombus than a ventilation–perfusion scan, and it can provide information on other potential causes of pulmonary symptoms.

4. Subsegmental emboli are often misdiagnosed on CT angiography.

Reference

Saad WE, Saad N. Computer tomography for venous thromboembolic disease. *Radiol Clin North Am.* 2007; 45:423-445.

Cross-Reference

Vascular and Interventional Radiology: THE REQUI-SITES, pp 198-207.

Comment

Although the clinical symptoms, electocardiographic findings, and chest radiography of patients with PE have been well characterized, these findings are nearly always nonspecific. Because the medical and procedural interventions for PE (e.g., anticoagulation and/or IVC filter placement) can have substantial morbidity, the diagnosis of pulmonary embolism requires imaging confirmation. Traditionally, ventilation–perfusion scanning has been used as the initial screening test for acute pulmonary embolism, but in recent years CT angiography has been investigated as a potentially superior screening examination.

To achieve optimal results with CTA, several factors must be present. There must be power IV injection of contrast into an arm vein at 3 to 5 mL/s. There must be helical scanning capability with reconstruction into small increments. There must be meticulous review of the scans by a radiologist with abundant experience in interpreting thoracic CT scans.

The sensitivity of multidetector CT scanning for detecting PE is 83% to 94%, with a specificity of 94% to 100% and a reader confidence of 90%. Furthermore, CT angiography provides a diagnosis of not PE in 70% of patients in whom PE was initially suspected but who were found not to have PE (>50% of patients in whom PE was initially suspected).

CASE 86

Hepatic Cirrhosis

1. Proper hepatic artery.

2. Corkscrew tortuosity of branch vessels.

3. Hepatic cirrhosis.

4. Increased.

Reference

Hori M, Murakami T, Kim T, et al. Diagnosis of hepatic neoplasms using CT arterial portography and CT hepatic arteriography. *Tech Vasc Interv Radiol.* 2002;5(3): 164-169.

Cross-Reference

Vascular and Interventional Radiology: THE REQUI-SITES, pp 608-615.

Comment

Arteriographic changes of cirrhosis are not typically apparent until there is substantial loss of liver parenchyma and the liver is fibrotic and contracted. Therefore, cirrhosis may be present long before the arteriographic changes are obvious. Early liver disease often results in hepatic swelling and enlargement, which can give a stretched appearance to the small arterial branches. As cirrhosis worsens and portal hypertension develops, portal venous return to the liver decreases. To compensate for this, hepatic arterial flow increases. This increased flow is the likely cause of these intrahepatic arterial changes. Ultimately, as fibrosis develops and worsens, the peripheral branches exhibit a characteristic corkscrew configuration. Occasionally, telangiectasias, aneurysms, or arterioportal venous shunting can be demonstrated.

Other vascular changes are notable in cirrhotic livers as well. The parenchymal phase of liver enhancement typically demonstrates a mottled appearance with nonuniform enhancement. Hypervascular masses within the parenchyma are highly suspicious for hepatocellular carcinoma. Portal venous flow can be hepatopedal or hepatofugal, and in some instances the portal vein can be occluded by thrombus or tumor.

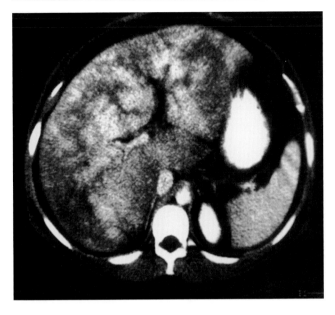 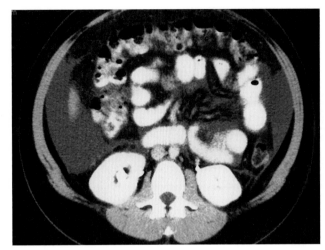

1. How can the definitive diagnosis of the hepatic pathology pictured above be obtained?

2. What factor visualized on the images would predispose this patient to complications of liver biopsy?

3. How would you obtain tissue from this liver if the patient's coagulation parameters were impaired?

4. How is this procedure performed?

C A S E 8 7

Transjugular Biopsy of Diffuse Liver Disease

1. Image-guided biopsy.

2. The presence of ascites.

3. Transjugular liver biopsy.

4. The right hepatic vein is selected and a biopsy needle is passed into the hepatic parenchyma using a metallic guiding cannula.

Reference

Wallace MJ, Narvios A, Lichtiger B, et al. Transjugular liver biopsy in patients with hematologic malignancy and severe thrombocytopenia. *J Vasc Interv Radiol*. 2003;14:323-327.

Cross-Reference

Vascular and Interventional Radiology: THE REQUI-SITES, pp 404-405.

Comment

In most patients with diffuse liver lesions, tissue diagnosis may be safely obtained by transabdominal percutaneous biopsy. However, patients with impaired coagulation and those with ascites are at significant risk for intraperitoneal bleeding following needle traversal of the liver capsule. Liver biopsy from a transjugular route is associated with a lower rate of bleeding complications and represents a safer option in these situations.

To perform transjugular liver biopsy, the right internal jugular vein is percutaneously accessed under ultrasound guidance. The right hepatic vein is selected and contrast venography may be used to confirm catheter position. The catheter is then exchanged for a metallic cannula. This cannula is directed anteriorly (away from the posterior liver capsule) under fluoroscopic guidance, and a specially designed long biopsy needle is used to obtain one or more core biopsy specimens from the hepatic parenchyma. If the middle hepatic vein is used instead of the right hepatic vein, then the cannula may be directed in a posterolateral direction to avoid the anterior liver capsule. The cannula is then removed and the jugular entry site is compressed for hemostasis. Hemostasis within the liver occurs quickly provided the hepatic capsule was not breached.

Notes

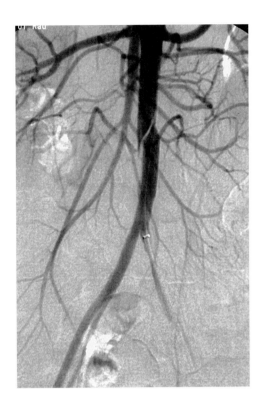
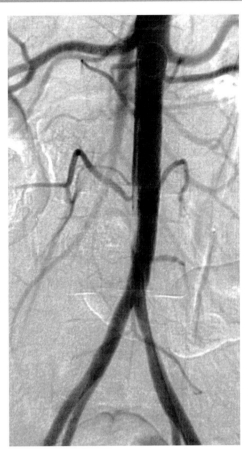

1. What abnormality is present in the first image?

2. What are the potential etiologies of this abnormality?

3. What treatment has been performed?

4. Are the indications for aortic stent placement different from those of iliac artery stent placement?

Iatrogenic Aortic Dissection

1. Abdominal aortic dissection.

2. Iatrogenic injury, trauma, hypertension, connective tissue disease.

3. Stent placement.

4. No.

Reference

Bariseel H, Batt M, Rogopoulos A, et al. Iatrogenic dissection of the abdominal aorta. *J Vasc Surg*. 1998; 27:366-370.

Cross-Reference

Vascular and Interventional Radiology: THE REQUISITES, pp 261-270.

Comment

The first image demonstrates a diagonally oriented intimal defect within the infrarenal abdominal aorta, consistent with a dissection flap. This patient had undergone angioplasty of a distal aortic stenosis 1 week earlier but did not experience improvement in her symptoms or in her femoral pulses.

The indications for bare stent placement in the abdominal aorta are identical to those for iliac artery stent placement: technical failure of percutaneous balloon angioplasty (>30% residual stenosis or >10 mm Hg systolic pressure gradient), recurrent stenosis following angioplasty, arterial dissection, and treatment of eccentric or heavily calcified stenoses.

Notes

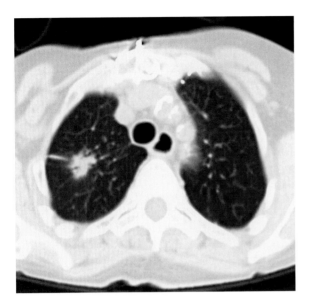

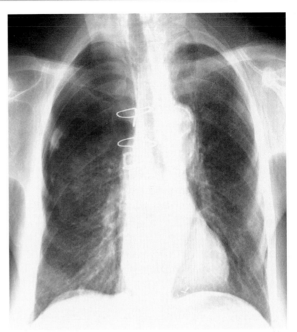

1. By what methods can a lung lesion be biopsied?

2. Can core biopsy be safely performed in the lung?

3. What complication of lung biopsy is visualized in the images?

4. Name two other complications of lung biopsy.

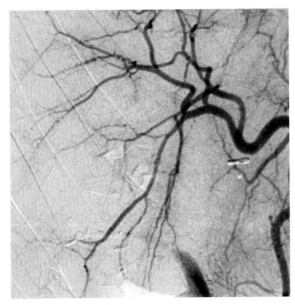

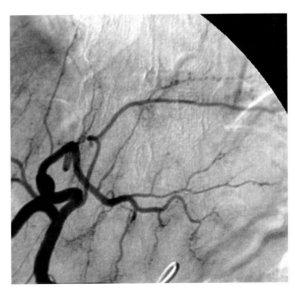

Courtesy of Dr. Daniel Brown.

Courtesy of Dr. Daniel Brown.

1. What is the most likely diagnosis?

2. Is the aorta likely to also be involved with this process?

3. Are the renal arteries likely to also be involved with this process?

4. Can these lesions be treated in endovascular fashion?

C A S E 8 9

CT-Guided Lung Biopsy with Pneumothorax

1. Percutaneous CT-guided, bronchoscopic, and surgical.

2. Yes.

3. Pneumothorax.

4. Hemothorax, severe hemoptysis.

Reference

Ohno Y, Hatabu H, Takenaka D, et al. CT-guided transthoracic needle aspiration biopsy of small solitary pulmonary nodules. *AJR Am J Roentenol.* 2003;180:1665-1669.

Cross-Reference

Vascular and Interventional Radiology: THE REQUISITES, pp 483-487.

Comment

Percutaneous lung biopsy is a safe procedure when performed by radiologists who are capable of managing its potential complications. For spiculated masses for which primary lung cancer is suspected, multiple fine-needle-aspiration specimens often suffice to make the diagnosis. For more complex lesions and when lymphoma is a diagnostic possibility, core biopsy is needed. Preprocedure planning should include careful evaluation of the CT scan and a review of the patient's overall cardiopulmonary status.

It is common (25%) for patients to experience a small amount of hemoptysis following the procedure, but massive hemoptysis and significant hemothorax are rare. Pneumothorax occurs in 15% to 30% of patients undergoing lung biopsy, but it only requires chest tube placement in 2% to 5%. Patients with chronic obstructive pulmonary disease, however, have a significantly higher risk of post-biopsy pneumothorax, with a more significant fraction requiring chest tube placement. In general, when chest tube placement is required, a small-bore tube (10-12 F) may be used and the tube can usually be removed within 1 to 3 days.

The incidence of pneumothorax may be reduced by the use of coaxial technique; by minimizing the number of pleural surfaces crossed by the needle, minimizing needle path length; and by avoiding oblique passes across pleural surfaces. A cytopathologist should be present to verify that sufficient tissue is obtained for confident diagnosis with a minimum number of needle passes.

C A S E 9 0

Polyarteritis Nodosa

1. Polyarteritis nodosa.

2. No.

3. Yes.

4. No.

Reference

Stanson AW, Friese JL, Johnson CM, et al. Polyarteritis nodosa: Spectrum of angiographic findings. *Radiographics.* 2001;21:151-159.

Cross-Reference

Vascular and Interventional Radiology: THE REQUISITES, p 320.

Comment

The images demonstrate multifocal irregularity, stenoses, and small aneurysms in the small and medium-sized arteries of the hepatic circulation. This appearance is most likely due to polyarteritis nodosa. Another condition that can produce an identical appearance is necrotizing angiitis due to drug abuse (often methamphetamines). When microaneurysms are present, the possibility of mycotic aneurysms must also be considered in the appropriate clinical context (e.g., fever and/or signs of sepsis), but the angiographic appearance shown here is much less likely to represent infection.

Polyarteritis nodosa is a systemic necrotizing vasculitis of small and medium-sized muscular arteries and arterioles. Patients can experience low-grade fever, myalgias and arthralgias, tender subcutaneous nodules, peripheral neuropathy, hematuria, and symptoms related to vascular involvement. The most commonly involved visceral vascular beds are the renal arteries (85%) and the hepatomesenteric circulation (50%). The large vessels, such as the aorta or major mesenteric trunks, are not likely to be involved.

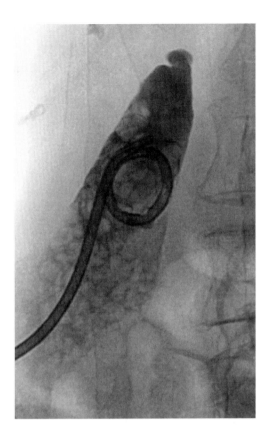

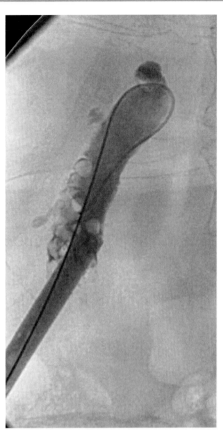

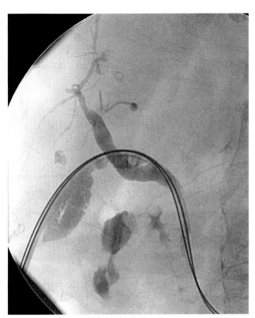

1. What procedure has been performed after the first image?

2. Is this procedure the treatment of choice for this condition?

3. Can the drainage catheter be removed immediately after the procedure?

4. Name two complications of this procedure.

Percutaneous Gallstone Removal

1. Percutaneous gallstone removal.

2. No. Surgical cholecystectomy is the treatment of choice.

3. No.

4. Bile peritonitis and sepsis.

Reference

Courtois CS, Picus D, Hicks ME. Percutaneous gallstone removal: Long-term follow-up. *J Vasc Intervent Radiol.* 1996;7:229-234.

Cross-Reference

Vascular and Interventional Radiology: THE REQUI-SITES, pp 597-601.

Comment

Patients with acute cholecystitis are often managed with catheter drainage during the initial phase. Once the acute infection and inflammation have resolved, a decision needs to be made as to what the appropriate definitive management should be. In most patients, surgical cholecystectomy should be performed, either using an open transabdominal approach or using laparoscopic technology.

Patients with significant contraindications for surgical resection are considered candidates for percutaneous methods of gallstone removal. After a mature transperitoneal tract has formed around the percutaneous cholecystostomy catheter (usually 2-4 weeks), the catheter is removed over a guidewire, the tract is dilated, and a large sheath is placed. Calculi are usually ultrasonically fragmented under endoscopic visualization, and the stone fragments are removed by aspiration and a variety of grasping devices. Following this, a drainage catheter is left in place. Once all stones are removed (as demonstrated by cholangiography), the cystic and common bile ducts are patent, and the patient is clinically well, the tube can be capped and subsequently removed.

The recurrence rate of gallstones following percutaneous removal is extremely high (perhaps 40% within 3 years). For this reason, this procedure is generally reserved for elderly patients with significant surgical contraindications.

Notes

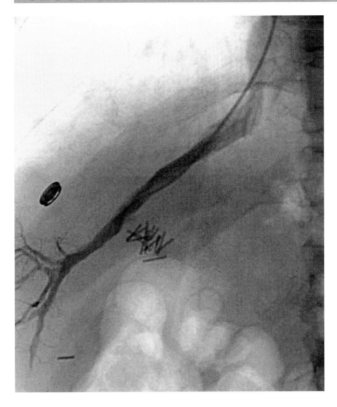

1. How has this study been performed?

2. Why might a balloon catheter be used diagnostically in this vein?

3. What major diagnosis can be made from hepatic vein pressure measurements?

4. Name two other reasons to catheterize this vein.

Hepatic Venography

1. The right hepatic vein has been selected from a jugular vein approach.

2. To obtain wedged hepatic vein pressures.

3. Portal hypertension.

4. To perform transjugular intrahepatic portosystemic shunt (TIPS); to evaluate for anatomic evidence of Budd–Chiari syndrome.

Reference

Pieters PC, Miller WJ, DeMeo JH. Evaluation of the portal venous system: Complementary roles of invasive and noninvasive imaging strategies. *Radiographics*. 1997;17:879-895.

Cross-Reference

Vascular and Interventional Radiology: THE REQUISITES, pp 399-401.

Comment

Hepatic vein catheterization is most easily accomplished from the right internal jugular vein, but it may also be performed from the left internal jugular vein or a femoral vein. The most common reasons to perform hepatic venography are to obtain pressure measurements to estimate the portal vein to systemic pressure gradient, to define the portal vein target site for TIPS via carbon dioxide portography, to perform the TIPS procedure, and to make the diagnosis of Budd–Chiari syndrome.

The corrected hepatic sinusoidal pressure is the difference between the wedged hepatic vein pressure (obtained with the balloon inflated and wedged distally) and the free hepatic vein pressure (the hepatic vein pressure obtained with the balloon deflated). The corrected hepatic sinusoidal pressure, which should be confirmed by measurement in at least two hepatic veins, provides a fairly accurate estimate of the portosystemic gradient except in the presence of severe parenchymal hepatic disease involving the presinusoidal venules. The normal corrected hepatic sinusoidal pressure is less than 5 mm Hg; a gradient greater than 6 mm Hg represents indirect evidence of portal hypertension, and a gradient of greater than 12 mm Hg is thought to correlate with an increased risk of variceal bleeding.

Notes

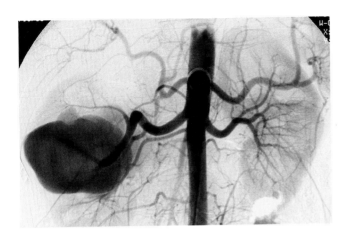

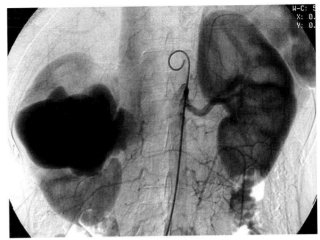

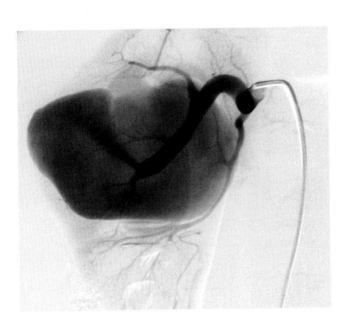

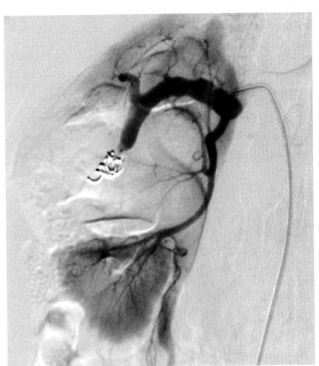

1. Describe the angiographic findings on the first two images.

2. Name three symptoms that may be present.

3. In this case, does the nidus require embolization?

4. In this case, is embolization likely to be a durable therapy?

Renal Arteriovenous Malformation

1. Enlarged right renal artery, arteriovenous malformation from a right renal artery branch vessel with early filling of the right renal vein and inferior vena cava.

2. Hematuria, hypertension, high-output cardiac failure.

3. No. This lesion is a simple arteriovenous fistula and no nidus is present.

4. Yes. This lesion has a single feeding vessel that can be embolized permanently.

Reference

Dinkel HP, Danauser H, Triller J. Blunt renal trauma: Minimally invasive management with microcatheter embolization experience in nine patients. *Radiology*. 2002;223:723-730.

Cross-Reference

Vascular and Interventional Radiology: THE REQUISITES, pp 346.

Comment

The selective right renal angiogram demonstrates opacification of a large arteriovenous malformation. Early filling of the venous system is a characteristic finding of such lesions and emphasizes the importance of considering whether all opacified structures are appropriate for the particular phase of the angiogram being evaluated. Opacification of venous structures should never be apparent on arterial phase images.

Renal arteriovenous malformations are rare lesions that may be congenital or acquired. When they are acquired, the most common cause is iatrogenic injury secondary to a renal biopsy or other intervention. The lesions often manifest with recurrent gross hematuria, and they can even produce renovascular hypertension. Successful endovascular treatment of the abnormality generally results in regression of these symptoms.

Endovascular therapy for simple renal arteriovenous malformations (like the one pictured here) usually consists of coil embolization of the feeding artery (as seen in the last image). If the lesion is more complex, then particle embolization may be used to treat the abnormality while preserving the kidney for as long as possible; however, such lesions often recur following embolization, and total or partial nephrectomy is likely to be needed eventually.

Notes

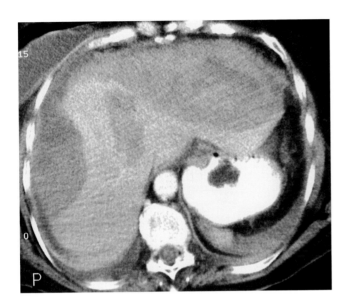

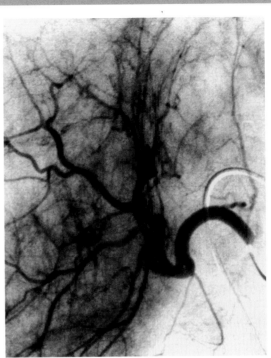

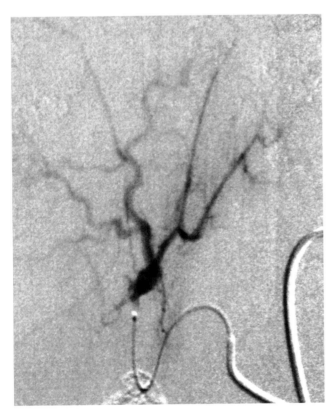

1. What abnormalities are seen on the images above?

2. What is the likely etiology?

3. What materials are commonly used for embolization in this setting?

4. What preprocedural CT findings would indicate a patient at higher risk for developing hepatic ischemia following embolization therapy?

Traumatic Hepatic Laceration

1. Two large subcapsular hematomas, a liver laceration, and a pseudoaneurysm arising from a left hepatic artery branch.

2. Trauma.

3. Coils and Gelfoam.

4. Portal vein thrombosis, other findings of severe portal hypertension including enlarged hepatic artery and the presence of varices.

Reference

Hagiwara A, Murata A, Matsuda T, et al. The efficacy and limitations of transarterial embolization for severe hepatic injury. *J Trauma*. 2002;52:1091-1096.

Cross-Reference

Vascular and Interventional Radiology: THE REQUI-SITES, pp 311-313.

Comment

Patients with blunt abdominal trauma are initially evaluated with contrast-enhanced CT scanning. Hepatic injuries are typically categorized on CT into five categories, and in many institutions patients with CT evidence of contrast extravasation and most patients with grade 3 to 5 injuries (grade 3 = laceration 3-10 cm in length or hematoma 3-10 cm in thickness) typically undergo arteriography to search for arterial bleeding. When bleeding is seen, embolization can be performed with a high likelihood of success.

Hepatic ischemia following embolization is common because approximately 70% of hepatic blood supply is derived from the portal venous system. For these reasons, when a laceration involves a large part of the hepatic parenchyma and multiple bleeding arteries are present, Gelfoam can be used to embolize an entire hepatic lobe rather than attempting to coil embolize each individual branch. However, patients with portal venous thrombosis and those with portal hypertension are at increased risk for hepatic ischemia, and embolization in these patients should be performed judiciously (portal hypertension patients) or not at all (portal vein thrombosis patients).

Notes

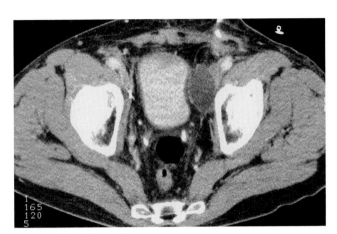

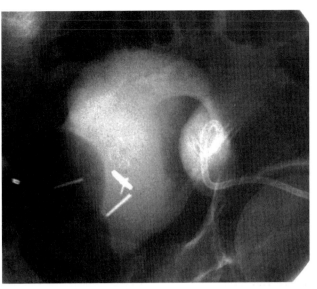

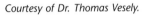

Courtesy of Dr. Thomas Vesely.

Courtesy of Dr. Thomas Vesely.

1. What abnormality is seen on the CT scan above?

2. What is the differential diagnosis in this patient who is status post pelvic lymph node dissection?

3. What laboratory studies should be performed on the aspirated fluid?

4. If persistently high drainage catheter outputs are seen several days after drainage and no fistula is present, does the patient require surgical management?

Pelvic Lymphocele

1. Left pelvic fluid collection.

2. Seroma, hematoma, urinoma, abscess, lymphocele.

3. Gram stain and bacterial culture, creatinine level, cell count, and differential.

4. No. The patient can undergo ethanol sclerosis if the lesion is a lymphocele.

Reference

Zuckerman DA, Yeager TD. Percutaneous ethanol sclerotherapy of postoperative lymphoceles. *AJR Am J Roentgenol.* 1997;169:433-437.

Cross-Reference

Vascular and Interventional Radiology: THE REQUISITES, pp 509-510.

Comment

The images demonstrate the typical appearance of a postoperative pelvic lymphocele. If the patient is symptomatic (commonly pain, fever, or leg swelling due to iliac vein compression), the intervention of first choice is percutaneous drainage.

The aspirated fluid should be sent for laboratory analysis as described, because the differential diagnosis is broad. If the collection is sterile and has an extremely high concentration of lymphocytes, the diagnosis of lymphocele is made.

Although catheter drainage is sometimes successful as stand-alone therapy, a significant percentage of lymphoceles do not completely resolve with catheter drainage alone because lymphatic channels within the wall of the collection continue to produce fluid. In this situation, if the collection is not infected and no fistula is present, then periodic (usually 2-3 times per week) instillation of absolute ethanol can produce cessation of fluid output from the collection, eventually allowing removal of the catheter. In general, at least several sessions of sclerosis are needed, and the entire process can take up to several months in a minority of cases.

Notes

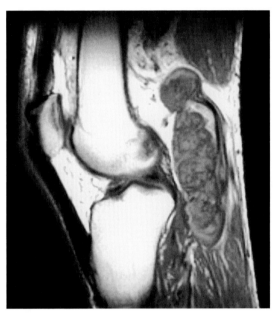

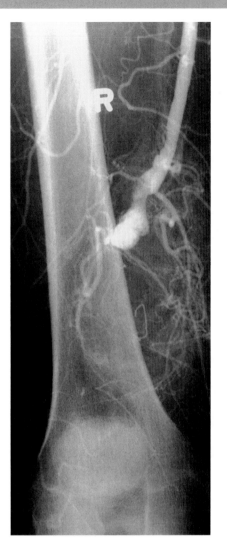

Courtesy of Dr. Thomas Vesely. *Courtesy of Dr. Thomas Vesely.*

1. What diagnosis is evident on the angiogram?

2. Is this likely to be an isolated lesion?

3. What complication of this lesion is apparent?

4. Is rupture a common complication of this lesion?

Popliteal Artery Aneurysm

1. Popliteal artery aneurysm.

2. No.

3. Popliteal artery thrombosis.

4. No.

Reference

Ascher E, Markevich N, Schutzer RW, et al. Small popliteal artery aneurysms: Are they clinically significant? *J Vasc Surg.* 2003;37:755-760.

Cross-Reference

Vascular and Interventional Radiology: THE REQUISITES, pp 435-436.

Comment

Popliteal artery aneurysms are commonly bilateral, and they often coexist with aneurysms in another location, most commonly abdominal aortic aneurysms and common femoral artery aneurysms. The most common presenting symptoms include lower-extremity ischemia and compression of adjacent nerves or other structures. Although rupture of popliteal aneurysms can occur, this complication is quite uncommon (<5% of patients). More commonly, popliteal aneurysms manifest with limb-threatening ischemia due to distal embolization (20%) or popliteal artery thrombosis (40%) (as seen in this case). Hence, even small aneurysms can produce limb-threatening ischemia.

The treatment of choice is surgical aneurysm resection with distal bypass. Stent grafts have been used to treat a small number of selected patients with popliteal artery aneurysms, but early stent-graft occlusion is very common. Hence, this approach can only be recommended for rare patients with very strong contraindications to surgical management.

Notes

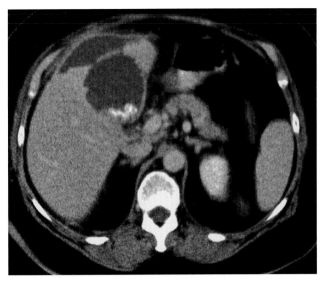

Courtesy of Dr. Thomas Vesely.

1. What is the diagnosis?

2. What is the etiology of this condition?

3. Does the visualized complication of this condition mandate immediate surgery?

4. What clinical criteria will be used to determine the timing of tube removal?

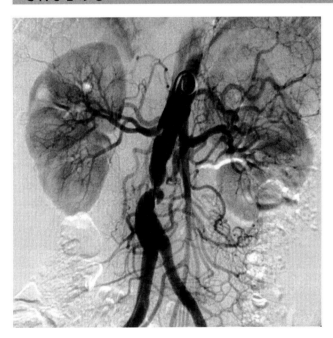

1. What symptoms are present in this female patient if the remainder of the lower extremity angiogram is normal?

2. What risk factor for atherosclerotic disease does this patient probably have?

3. Is this lesion likely to respond to angioplasty?

4. Does the patient require anticoagulation following percutaneous intervention with a good technical result?

Gallbladder Rupture with Pericholecystic Abscess

1. Acute cholecystitis with gallbladder rupture and pericholecystic abscess formation.

2. Gallstones with subsequent cystic duct obstruction.

3. No. Percutaneous cholecystostomy can still be performed provided the pericholecystic abscess is drained, too.

4. The tube remains in place until surgical gallbladder resection is performed. Alternatively, if percutaneous gallstone removal is performed, the tube should remain in place until a mature tract is present around the tube, no residual gallstones are seen, the cystic and common bile ducts are patent, and the patient is clinically well, with the tube capped.

Reference

Ahkan O, Akinsi D, Ozmen MN. Percutaneous cholecystostomy. *Eur J Radiol*. 2002;43(3):229-236.

Cross-Reference

Vascular and Interventional Radiology: THE REQUISITES, pp 593-597.

Comment

Complications of acute cholecystitis can include free rupture into the peritoneum or contained rupture with pericholecystic abscess formation. Historically, the presence of gallbladder rupture was an absolute indication for emergency cholecystectomy. In modern practice, however, most surgeons much prefer to operate after the acute infection and pericholecystic inflammation have subsided. For these reasons, percutaneous cholecystostomy may still be performed. However, the abscess must also be drained, either using the same drainage catheter with additional side holes created to drain the abscess (as was done in this case) or via a separate (second) catheter.

Abdominal Aortic Stenosis

1. Bilateral hip and buttock claudication.

2. Smoking history.

3. Yes.

4. No.

Reference

Sandhu C, Belli AM. Abdominal aortic stenting: Current practice. *Abdom Imaging*. 2001;6:453-460.

Cross-Reference

Vascular and Interventional Radiology: THE REQUISITES, pp 261-270.

Comment

Although hypertension, diabetes, and hyperlipidemia are all associated with the development of atherosclerotic lesions, patients with a history of smoking are particularly prone to develop occlusive disease in the aorta and iliac arteries. Although aortofemoral bypass grafting is associated with high patency rates, percutaneous interventions are usually used first for appropriate lesions because of their lower morbidity rates.

Invasive therapy is only performed in patients with lifestyle–limiting claudication or rest pain. For focal, concentric, short lesions (as in this case), percutaneous balloon angioplasty is an appropriate first treatment. Patencies following aortic angioplasty are comparable to those associated with iliac artery lesions.

Postangioplasty stent placement may be performed if flow–limiting dissection occurs following angioplasty, if angioplasty fails to reduce the stenosis to less than 30% diameter, if a persistent pressure gradient (>10 mm Hg systolic) is present across the lesion after angioplasty, or if the stenosis recurs following successful angioplasty. Primary stent placement (placement of a stent without preceding angioplasty) is generally used for extremely calcified or eccentric lesions.

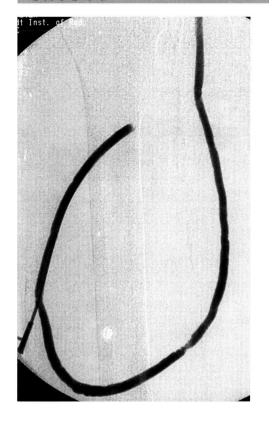

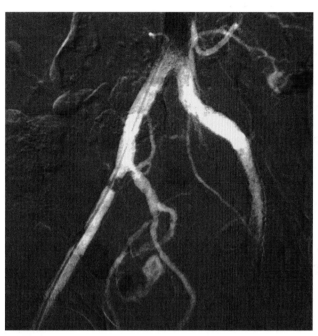

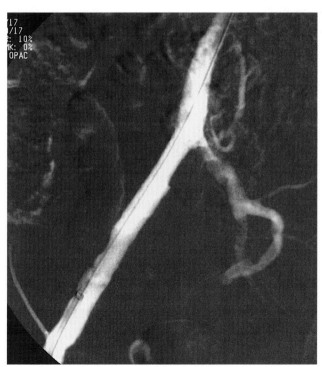

1. What diagnostic study has been performed and why?

2. Assuming that the iliac and common femoral veins are normal, what is the cause of the low flows seen in this patient?

3. How often is arterial inflow the major factor in hemodialysis graft malfunction?

4. What is the most common anatomic cause of hemodialysis graft malfunction or occlusion?

Iliac Artery Stenosis Above a Hemodialysis Graft

1. Right femoral dialysis fistulogram was performed to evaluate the cause of hemodialysis graft malfunction.

2. Right external iliac artery stenosis.

3. From 5% to 10% of cases.

4. Stenosis at the venous anastomosis.

Reference

Surlan M, Popovic P. The role of interventional radiology in management of patients with end-stage renal disease. *Eur J Radiol.* 2003;46(2):96-114.

Cross-Reference

Vascular and Interventional Radiology: THE REQUISITES, pp 184-191.

Comment

Although hemodialysis grafts are most often placed in the upper extremity, the presence of central venous occlusion with subsequent graft failure often necessitates a search for alternative access sites. The common femoral veins are usually used for dialysis access, but they are prone to the same complications as upper-extremity dialysis access.

The vast majority of culprit stenoses occur at the venous anastomosis of the graft, within the graft, within the peripheral or central venous outflow veins, or at the arterial anastomosis. However, when the angiographic appearance of these regions does not explain the clinical findings of graft malfunction, then the entire arterial inflow to the graft should be studied arteriographically. When a culprit stenosis is identified, treatment with angioplasty or stent placement (as seen in the last image) may be performed.

Notes

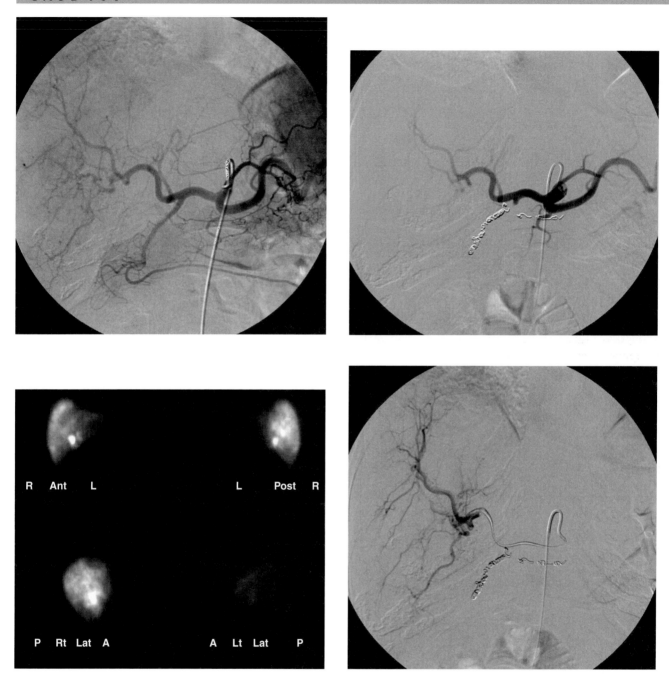

1. Which artery is being selectively injected on the first image?

2. Which arteries have been selectively embolized on the second image?

3. Name the radiotracer used to obtain the images in the third image.

4. Name the radioisotope used for treatment of this patient with metastatic colorectal cancer in the fourth image.

Colorectal Metastases to Liver: Radioembolization

1. Celiac axis.

2. Gastroduodenal and right gastric arteries.

3. Technetium-99m macroaggregated albumin (^{99m}Tc-MAA).

4. Yttrium-90 microspheres (^{90}Y microspheres).

Reference

Salem R, Thurston KG. Radioembolization with ^{90}Yttrium microspheres: A state-of-the-art brachytherapy treatment for primary and secondary liver malignancies. Part 1: Technical and methodologic considerations. *J Vasc Interv Radiol*. 2006;17:1251-1278.

Comment

Radioembolization with ^{90}Y microspheres is an FDA-approved therapy for treating unresectable hepatocellular carcinoma and metastatic colorectal carcinoma to the liver. The microspheres are delivered to the tumors in a transcatheter approach through the hepatic artery and, once in place, emit radiation that acts on the tumor cells. Careful patient selection is necessary to obtain optimal results. Owing to the variation in hepatic arterial anatomy and the potential complications that can result from nontarget embolization of microspheres to the bowel, gallbladder, pancreas, and other nearby structures that derive part of their arterial supply from branches closely associated with those that supply the liver, careful mapping of the arterial supply to the intended target lesion(s) and optimization of the arterial anatomy by selective embolization of vessels is mandatory.

After optimizing the arterial anatomy, the microcatheter tip is placed in the planned position for delivery of the radioembolic microspheres and approximately 5 mCi of ^{99m}Tc-MAA is delivered through the microcatheter. This is followed by CT SPECT imaging to assess the activity within the liver and to detect any activity in extrahepatic abdominal structures and the lungs to evaluate for nontarget delivery and tumor arteriovenous shunting, respectively.

Once the planning images are reviewed and the patient is deemed a candidate for treatment, dosimetry data are calculated. Dosimetry calculation methods vary; however, some factors that are considered include body surface area, liver volume, tumor burden, and underlying liver cirrhosis. The dose delivery must be carefully monitored under fluoroscopy to ensure that stasis is not reached.

Notes

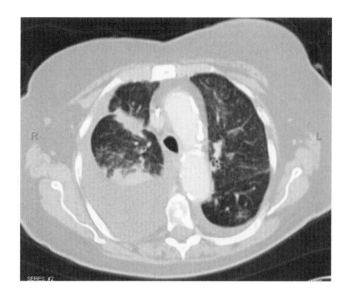

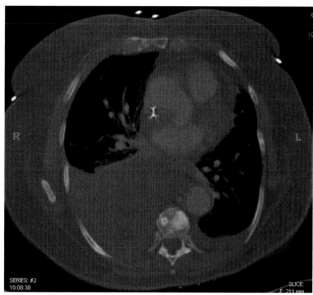

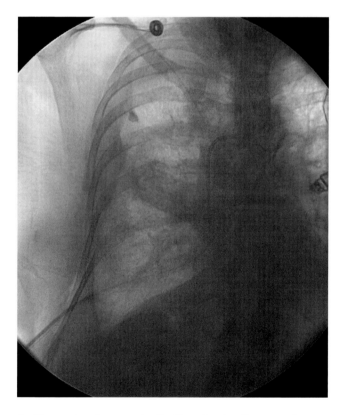

1. Name the three main findings in the first two images.

2. What is the diagnosis?

3. What procedure has been performed in the third image?

4. What symptom is likely to be relieved by this procedure?

Malignant Pleural Effusion: Tunneled Pleural Catheter Placement

1. Spiculated right lung mass, large right pleural effusion, and vertebral body metastases.

2. Metastatic lung cancer.

3. Placement of a tunneled pleural catheter (TPC).

4. Dyspnea.

References

Pollak JS, Burdge CM, Rosenblatt M, et al. Treatment of malignant pleural effusions with tunneled long-term drainage catheters. *J Vasc Interv Radiol*. 2001;12: 201-208.

Pollak JS. Malignant pleural effusions: Treatment with tunneled long-term drainage catheters. *Curr Opin Pulm Med*. 2002;8:302-307.

Comment

Pleural effusions often complicate the course of malignant disease and are poor prognostic indicators. The impact on patients' quality of life is significant, and the most common symptom is dyspnea. The approach to management is a palliative one and has traditionally been by thoracostomy and pleurodesis. More recently, management has been trending toward minimally invasive procedures by placement of TPCs.

Ultrasound or fluoroscopic guidance is used for accessing the pleural cavity, and the catheter is placed through a peel-away sheath and subsequently tunneled in the subcutaneous tissues of the chest. The catheter has a one-way valve that prevents leakage of pleural fluid from the catheter when it is not connected to a drainage flask and also prevents the entry of air into the pleural cavity through the catheter.

Ninety percent of patients experience relief of dyspnea within 48 hours. Spontaneous pleurodesis can occur in up to 46% of patients, usually within a month of placement. Chemical sclerotherapy through the catheter can be used to increase the rate of pleurodesis. If pleurodesis is achieved, the catheter may be removed.

Notes

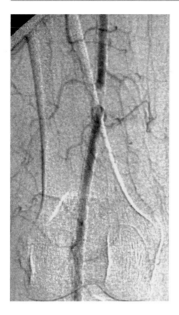
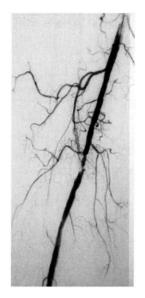
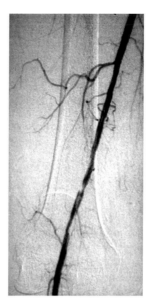

1. Name three methods of treating the lesion seen in the first image.

2. What has probably been done between the first and second images?

3. Describe the findings on the final image, which was obtained after angioplasty.

4. Is this an abnormal physiologic response to angioplasty?

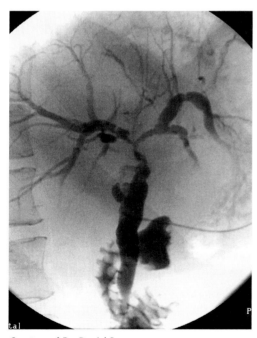
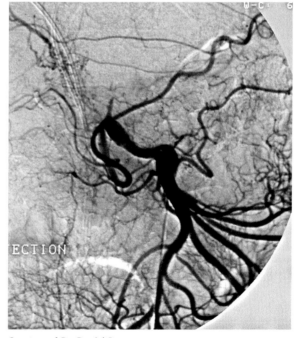

Courtesy of Dr. Daniel Brown.   *Courtesy of Dr. Daniel Brown.*

1. What abnormality is present in the biliary system of this liver transplant patient?

2. What is the likely etiology?

3. How would this be managed?

4. If the arterial problem was stenosis rather than occlusion, could angioplasty be performed?

Iatrogenic Superficial Femoral Artery Dissection

1. Femoropopliteal bypass, thrombolysis with subsequent angioplasty (this was done in this case), primary stent placement.

2. Thrombolysis.

3. Extensive arterial dissection, which is likely to limit flow.

4. Not really. The primary mechanism by which angioplasty works is via creation of controlled intimal dissection.

Reference

Lipsitz EC, Ohki T, Veith FJ, et al. Does subintimal angioplasty have a role in the treatment of severe lower extremity ischemia? *J Vasc Surg.* 2003;37:386-391.

Cross-Reference

Vascular and Interventional Radiology: THE REQUISITES, pp 419-428.

Comment

Repeat angiography is always performed immediately following angioplasty in order to assess whether the stenosis has been adequately treated and to evaluate for any complications. It is wise to perform angiography in two projections because intimal dissection flaps oriented in the coronal plane might not be appreciated on a single anteroposterior view. Postangioplasty pressure measurements across the lesion may also be obtained: If an unexplained significant (>10 mm Hg) systolic pressure gradient is still present, the presence of occult dissection should be suspected. Intravascular ultrasound, when available, can be extremely helpful in clarifying whether this is indeed the case and in assessing the entire extent of the dissection process.

Dissections caused by retrograde passage of a guidewire in a false channel often resolve spontaneously. Anterograde dissections are more likely to extend and to occlude flow.

Flow-limiting dissections require urgent treatment to prevent thrombosis. Most iliac artery dissections that do not extend into the common femoral artery can be managed with stent placement. Because patency rates for superficial femoral artery stents are comparatively poor, surgical bypass may be a better choice if the patient is thought to be able to tolerate a surgical procedure.

Hepatic Artery Thrombosis with Biliary Strictures

1. Extensive stricturing of the central biliary ducts.

2. Ischemia due to hepatic artery thrombosis.

3. Surgical revascularization of the arterial supply to the transplant, and biliary drainage.

4. Yes.

Reference

Saad WE, Saad NE, Davies MG, et al. Transhepatic balloon dilation of anastomotic biliary strictures in liver transplant recipients: The significance of a patent hepatic artery. *J Vasc Interv Radiol.* 2005;16:1221-1228.

Cross-Reference

Vascular and Interventional Radiology: THE REQUISITES, pp 580-584.

Comment

In the case shown, tight stricturing of the right and left central biliary ducts is evident on cholangiography, and the angiogram demonstrates thrombosis of the transplant hepatic artery that was anastomosed to a native replaced right hepatic artery.

A variety of anatomic complications can occur in patients who have undergone liver transplantation: biliary anstomotic leak, stenosis of the biliary anastomosis, stenosis at the inferior vena caval anastomosis, and hepatic artery anastomotic stenosis with subsequent thrombosis. Patients who experience hepatic artery thrombosis are prone to develop biliary strictures and/or necrosis. When this occurs, the strictures are usually centrally located and may be quite extensive and irregular in appearance.

Patients with evidence of transplant malfunction usually undergo sonographic evaluation. When elevated velocities are observed near the arterial anastomosis, a stenosis is suspected and the patient is usually referred for confirmatory angiography. Angioplasty can be performed to treat such stenoses, or surgical anastomotic revision may be performed. When hepatic artery thrombosis is present, surgical therapy is needed.

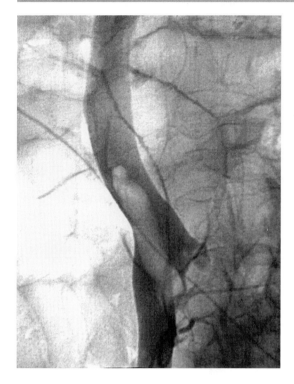

1. Is this abnormality acute or chronic?

2. If the patient has no contraindication to anticoagulation, should an inferior vena cava (IVC) filter be placed anyway?

3. If an IVC filter is being placed, what access site should be used?

4. Has catheter-directed thrombolysis been shown to be a better treatment for this problem?

C A S E 1 0 4

Free-Floating Inferior Vena Cava Thrombus

1. Acute.

2. Yes.

3. Right internal jugular vein (best choice) or left common femoral vein.

4. Not yet. However, if the patient has no contraindications to thrombolysis and is reasonably healthy otherwise, catheter-directed thrombolysis probably does offer a lower risk of later developing post-phlebitic symptoms.

Reference

Proctor MC. Indications for filter placement. *Semin Vasc Surg.* 2000;13(3):194-198.

Cross-Reference

Vascular and Interventional Radiology: THE REQUI-SITES, pp 361-368.

Comment

The images demonstrate a large ovoid filling defect within the right iliac vein extending into the inferior vena cava, consistent with a large free-floating acute thrombus. The venographic appearance of this abnormality suggests a predilection for easy migration and embolization. This necessitates extreme care if catheter manipulations are performed in this region, either for IVC filter placement or for thrombolytic therapy. Free-floating iliac vein and/or IVC thrombus is considered an indication for filter placement, even if no other contraindications to anticoagulation exist.

Notes

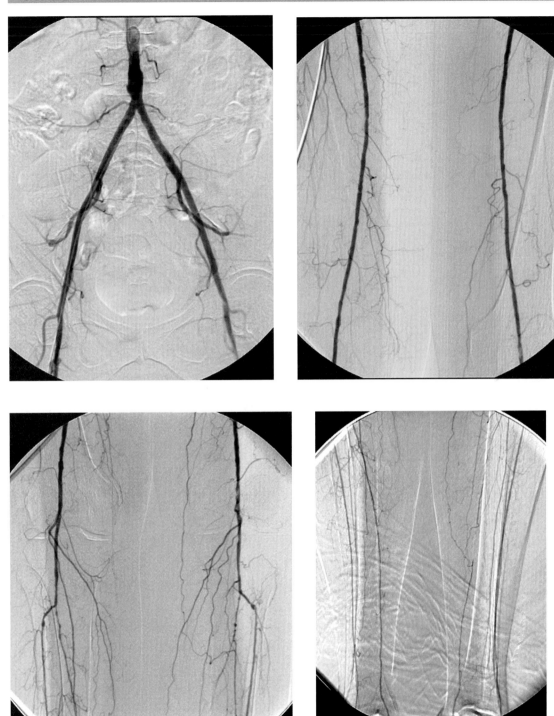

1. What are the primary findings of the angiogram depicted above?

2. What is the probable cause of the observed abnormalities?

3. What surgical treatment might be performed in such a patient?

4. What endovascular options exist for this patient?

Diabetes-Related Tibial Atherosclerosis

1. Bilateral occlusion of the posterior tibial arteries and severe stenosis of the peroneal arteries.

2. Diabetes mellitus.

3. Femoral–distal arterial bypass graft placement.

4. None.

Reference

Kellicut III DC, Sidawy AN, Arora S. Diabetic vascular disease and its management. *Semin Vasc Surg.* 2003; 16(1):12-18.

Cross-Reference

Vascular and Interventional Radiology: THE REQUI-SITES, pp 419-425.

Comment

Although smoking, hypertension, and hyperlipidemia also promote atherosclerosis, a particular pattern of arterial involvement is often seen in patients with diabetes mellitus. The primary feature of this pattern is multifocal severe stenoses and/or occlusions of the distal popliteal artery, tibioperoneal trunk, and the proximal segments of the anterior tibial, posterior tibial, and peroneal arteries. This typical pattern of disease often occurs in the presence of normal or near-normal iliac and femoral arteries in diabetic patients, as seen in the images here, although diabetic patients are certainly prone to atherosclerotic lesions in the more proximal arteries.

The clinical manifestations of diabetic arteriopathy are often more severe than the angiogram might indicate, because of the presence of microvascular disease not appreciated on angiography. Because patients with diabetic neuropathy are prone to pedal trauma, the combination of arterial insufficiency and trauma leads to frequent ulceration with difficulty in healing. Surgical arterial revascularization is commonly performed to help with ulcer healing in these patients. Unfortunately, limb amputation owing to vascular insufficiency is a fairly common event in this patient subset.

Notes

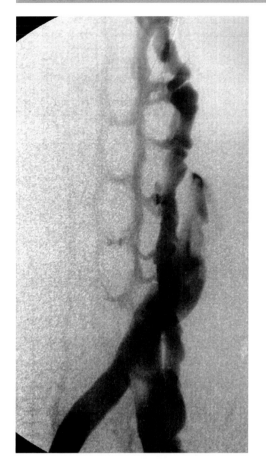
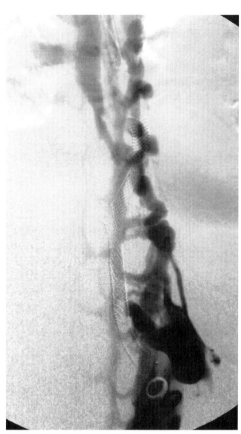

1. What is the primary abnormality?

2. Is this finding acute or chronic?

3. What symptoms might this patient have?

4. What vascular systems are serving as collateral networks?

Chronic Inferior Vena Cava Occlusion

1. Chronic inferior vena cava (IVC) occlusion.

2. Chronic.

3. Resting or ambulatory lower-extremity edema, venous claudication, lower-extremity hyperpigmentation and/or ulcerations.

4. Lumbar venous plexus and azygos/hemiazygos system.

Reference

Razavi MK, Hansch EC, Kee ST, et al. Chronically occluded inferior venae cavae: Endovascular treatment. *Radiology*. 2000;214:133-138.

Cross-Reference

Vascular and Interventional Radiology: THE REQUISITES, pp 361-364.

Comment

The images demonstrate occlusion of the distal IVC and reconstitution of the suprarenal IVC by collaterals from the lumbar venous plexus and azygos and hemiazygos system. Given the prominent visualization of the collateral network, the occlusion has undoubtedly been present for at least a few weeks and possibly years. Occlusion of the IVC can be caused by extension of iliofemoral deep vein thrombosis, IVC filters, and abdominal masses.

Patients with chronic IVC occlusion are typically treated with anticoagulation and lower-extremity compression stockings. Although this management is generally sufficient to prevent pulmonary embolism in all but a few cases, these patients tend to experience severe long-term post-thrombotic symptoms. For this reason, in carefully selected patients with severe symptoms, aggressive endovascular therapy may be attempted. Aggressive endovascular therapy consists of stent placement with a course of preceding thrombolysis if any acute thrombus is thought to be present.

Notes

Challenge

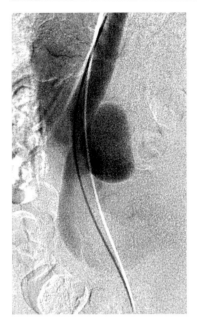 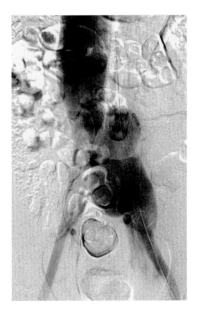

1. What vessels are abnormally opacified on this nonselective pelvic angiogram?

2. What vascular abnormality is seen on the oblique image?

3. Is this patient likely to be symptomatic?

4. What treatment options are considered for this type of problem?

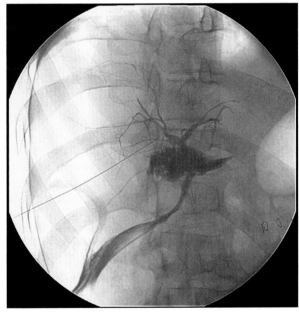 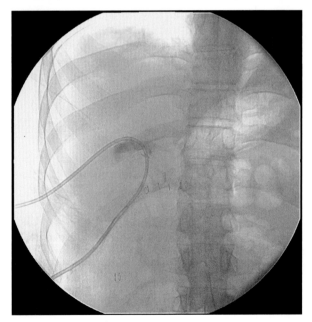

Courtesy of Dr. Daniel Brown. *Courtesy of Dr. Daniel Brown.*

1. What problem is visualized in the first image?

2. Name two likely potential etiologies for this problem.

3. Is immediate percutaneous biliary drainage the best initial treatment option?

4. What biliary ductal variant is important to consider in patients presenting with postoperative bile leaks?

CASE 107

Aortocaval Fistula

1. The left iliac vein and the inferior vena cava (IVC).

2. Pseudoaneurysm of the aortic bifurcation with a fistula to the IVC.

3. Yes.

4. Surgical ligation of the fistula with arterial repair, insertion of a stent graft, ligation or embolization of the artery distal and proximal to the fistula site with subsequent femorofemoral bypass grafting (not an option in the case above).

Reference

Parodi JC, Schonholz C, Ferreira LM, et al. Endovascular surgical treatment of traumatic arterial lesions. *Ann Vasc Surg*. 1999;13(2):121-129.

Cross-Reference

Vascular and Interventional Radiology: THE REQUI-SITES, pp 442-443.

Comment

The images demonstrate an aortic bifurcation pseudo-aneurysm with formation of a fistulous connection to the common iliac vein confluence.

Arteriovenous fistulas can occur as congenital abnormalities or as rare complications of trauma and surgery. Clinical manifestations can include high-output cardiac failure, ischemia distal to the fistula due to steal, dilated and enlarged peripheral veins, stasis dermatitis and ulceration due to increased venous pressure distal to the fistula, swelling of distal tissues, a palpable mass, an audible bruit, and a palpable thrill.

Angiography is useful to confirm the diagnosis of an arteriovenous fistula and delineate the anatomy, including the site of the fistula, its relationship to the involved vessels, and the presence of nearby branches that would confound endovascular repair. Large-volume injections in multiple projections with rapid filming are often necessary owing to the high flow volumes. Depending upon the location of the fistula and the presence of regional side branches, stent-graft placement can be used to seal the defect in patients who are poor candidates for surgery on anatomic or medical grounds.

CASE 108

Common Hepatic Duct Transection

1. Common hepatic duct transection with biloma formation.

2. Iatrogenic injury during laparoscopic cholecystectomy, and trauma.

3. Not necessarily. Biloma drainage is often a better and easier initial step.

4. Aberrant right posterior duct.

Reference

Saad N, Darcy M. Iatrogenic bile duct injury during laparoscopic cholecystectomy. *Tech Vasc Interv Radiol*. 2008;11:102-110.

Cross-Reference

Vascular and Interventional Radiology: THE REQUI-SITES, pp 579-580.

Comment

Bile duct injury is a dreaded complication of laparoscopic or open cholecystectomy, because in these situations, patients often require multiple radiologic interventions and/or complex surgical repair. The images here demonstrate contrast extravasating from the common hepatic duct and collecting as a biloma in the right subhepatic space and paracolic gutter. The distal common bile duct is not visualized, indicating a complete ductal transection.

The rate of technical failure of percutaneous biliary drainage is less than 5% in patients with dilated biliary ducts, but it can be as high as 25% in patients without ductal dilation. For this reason, in cases of major ductal injury, a percutaneous drainage catheter may first be placed within the easily accessible biloma to obtain initial control of the leak. After several weeks to a few months, a mature tract might form between the collapsed biloma cavity and the site of ductal injury. At this time, contrast injected into the biloma drain can opacify the biliary system, facilitating biliary drainage. In many cases, passage of a guidewire into the bowel is not possible; in these patients, a snare catheter may be used from the biloma access site to externalize the biliary wire and enable placement of a U-tube (second image), which is more stable than an external biliary drainage catheter. The presence of a drainage catheter assists the surgeon in identifying the duct during dissection, because there may be significant inflammation within the hepatic hilum. Ultimately, definitive surgical repair with hepaticojejunostomy is usually performed.

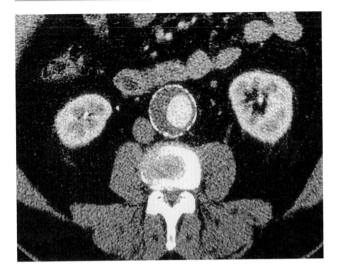 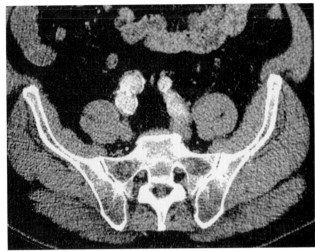

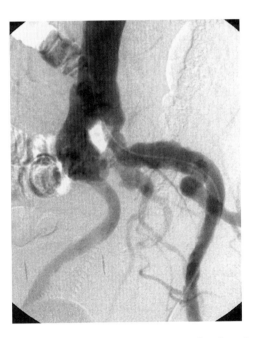 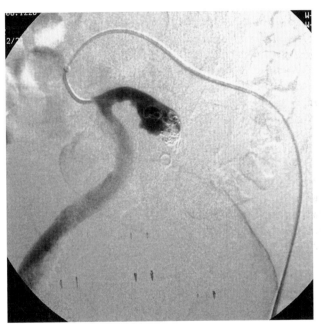

1. Describe the major finding in the first three images.

2. What treatment options exist for this problem?

3. What procedure was performed before the final image and why?

4. What significant clinical sequelae might this procedure produce?

Internal Iliac Artery Embolization

1. Abdominal aortic aneurysm (AAA) extending into the right common iliac artery.

2. Surgical repair of an aneurysm or placement of a stent graft if the aneurysm is large enough to warrant treatment (generally 5 cm, although 4-cm AAAs are treated by some).

3. Right internal iliac artery embolization, to prevent endoleak resulting from cross-pelvic collateral flow following stent-graft repair.

4. Ipsilateral buttock claudication and/or pelvic or colonic ischemia.

Reference

Cynamon J, Lerer D, Veith FJ, et al. Hypogastric artery coil embolization prior to endoluminal repair of aneurysms and fistulas: Buttock claudication, a recognized but possibly preventable complication. *J Vasc Intervent Radiol.* 2000;11:573-577.

Cross-Reference

Vascular and Interventional Radiology: THE REQUISITES, pp 252-261.

Comment

A variety of anatomic issues must be addressed before placing a stent graft for AAA. First, the iliac arteries must be of suitable caliber (7–8 mm) to permit introduction of the stent-graft delivery apparatus. Second, the proximal and distal necks of the aneurysm should be of sufficient length (>15 mm) and diameter (device-specific but usually <26-30 mm), and should be free of significant angulation or plaque, which can interfere with proper seating of the device. Third, the distance from the origin of the lowest renal artery to the origin of the internal iliac artery must be measured in order to select the proper device length.

When AAA involves the common iliac artery and the distal neck measures less than 15 mm, the potential exists for late aneurysm rupture due to endoleak via cross-pelvic collaterals from the contralateral internal iliac artery. For this reason, ipsilateral internal iliac artery coil embolization is performed to prevent this. Two main postprocedural adverse sequelae exist: First, if the contralateral internal iliac artery and inferior mesenteric artery are severely diseased, colonic ischemia can result. Second, about 40% of patients experience buttock claudication after internal iliac artery embolization; although this resolves spontaneously in two thirds of patients within a year, it can be a lifestyle-limiting long-term problem in a minority of patients. The problems can be prevented to some degree by embolizing only the main trunk of the internal iliac artery and not its branches.

Notes

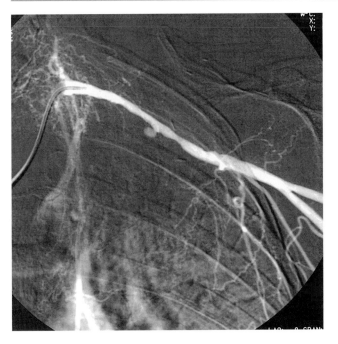
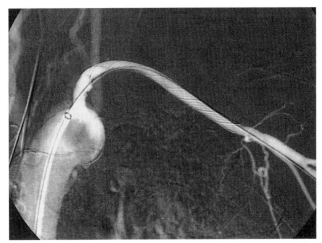

1. What study has been performed in the first image in this acutely bleeding patient with metastatic nodal disease in the left axilla?

2. What angiographic finding in the first image would explain the clinical findings?

3. What procedure has been performed before the second image?

4. Is this likely to represent a durable solution to this problem?

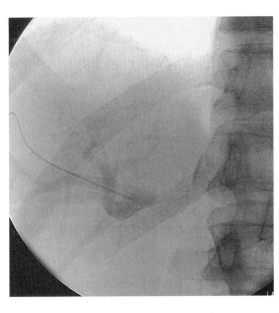
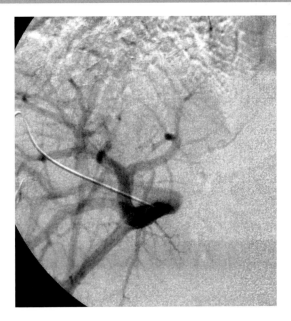

1. What vessel is being injected in the images above?

2. Why might this examination have been performed?

3. Name two major potential complications of this procedure.

4. How often is the portal vein bifurcation extrahepatic?

CASE 110

Axillary Artery Stent-Graft Placement

1. Selective left subclavian arteriogram.

2. Pseudoaneurysm from the left axillary artery.

3. Stent-graft placement in the left axillary artery.

4. No. This procedure is palliative. Recurrent bleeding and/or stent-graft occlusion represent potential future problems.

Reference

Hilfiker PR, Razavi MK, Kee ST, et al. Stent-graft therapy for subclavian artery aneurysms and fistulas: Single-center mid-term results. *J Vasc Intervent Radiol.* 2000;11:578-584.

Cross-Reference

Vascular and Interventional Radiology: THE REQUISITES, pp 158-159.

Comment

In this case, hypervascularity is observed within the lower neck, consistent with the history of metastatic disease. A small pseudoaneurysm arises from the left axillary artery. Given the patient's short life expectancy and the presence of tumor in this area, surgical repair would be undesirable and maybe impossible. For this reason, a stent graft was percutaneously inserted across the pseudoaneurysm, providing hemostasis.

The use of nonaortic stent grafts is increasing. Because the long-term durability of these devices has not yet been established, careful patient selection criteria must be used. However, this technology often enables treatment of very difficult surgical problems in a minimally invasive manner.

The stent component of a stent graft enables enlargement of a vascular lumen and facilitates graft fixation. The graft component of the stent graft enables one to reline the interior of a vessel wall. Current applications for these devices include: (1) Atherosclerosis: the graft lining is thought to be associated with lower restenosis potential than bare stents; (2) Peripheral aneurysms; (3) Trauma-related vascular injury in patients with high surgical risk; (4) Arteriovenous fistulas and similar lesions.

CASE 111

Portal Vein Access for Islet Cell Transplantation

1. Right portal vein.

2. To guide a transjugular intrahepatic portosystemic shunt (TIPS) or to perform islet cell transplantation in diabetic patients.

3. Portal vein thrombosis and intraperitoneal hemorrhage.

4. Approximately 50% of patients.

References

Lin J, Zhou KR, Chen ZW, et al. 3D contrast-enhanced MR portography and direct x-ray portography: A correlation study. *Eur Radiol.* 2003;12:1277-1285.

Goss JA, Soltes G, Goodpastor SE, et al. Pancreatic islet transplantation: The radiographic approach. *Transplantation.* 2003;76:199-203.

Cross-Reference

Vascular and Interventional Radiology: THE REQUISITES, pp 383-386.

Comment

Direct portography via percutaneous catheter placement in the right portal vein for infusion of islet cells in a diabetic patient is depicted. Although this particular procedure is still investigational, direct portal vein access can be useful in a few clinical situations. When estimation of portal pressures is confounded by the presence of sinusoidal liver disease, a small catheter may be placed in the portal vein for direct pressure transduction. When transjugular portal vein access during TIPS is thought to be challenging, some physicians place a catheter within the right portal vein to provide a target for transhepatic puncture. In carefully selected patients, the percutaneous route may be used to clear thrombus from a thrombosed portal vein before placing a TIPS.

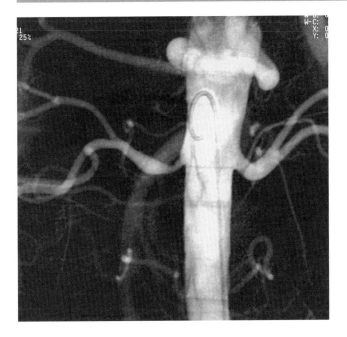
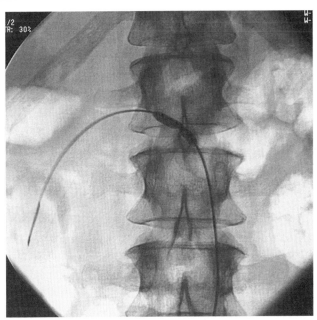
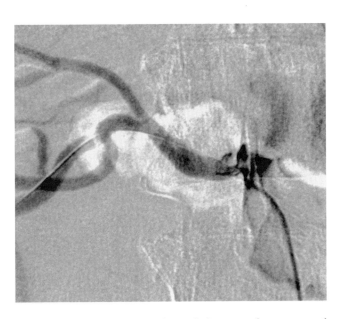
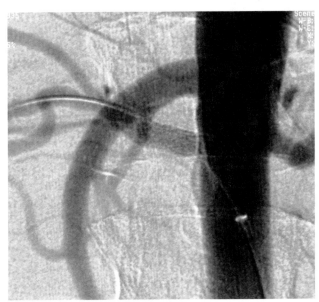

1. What is the minimum desired diameter for a stent placed in a renal artery?

2. How may stenosis in a small renal artery be treated?

3. If percutaneous and surgical revascularization are not possible owing to the small vessel size, what procedure can be used to ameliorate renovascular hypertension?

4. If it is unclear from angiography and scintigraphy whether a stenosis is causing renovascular hypertension, what procedure may be performed to clarify this?

Stenosis in a Small Renal Artery

1. Below 6 mm the significance of even mild degrees of intimal hyperplasia is great. Stent placement is not likely to lead to durable success in small vessels.

2. Percutaneous transluminal angioplasty, aortorenal bypass.

3. A renal artery supplying only a small amount of parenchyma may be embolized and that parenchyma sacrificed to treat renovascular hypertension.

4. Renal vein renin sampling.

Reference

Martin LG, Cork RD, Wells JO. Renal vein renin analysis: Limitations in predicting benefit for percutaneous angioplasty. *Cardiovasc Intervent Radiol.* 1993;16:76-80.

Cross-Reference

Vascular and Interventional Radiology: THE REQUISITES, pp 327-336.

Comment

The images depict a stenosis in a fairly small renal artery. A poor technical result was observed after angioplasty (third image), so a stent was placed. The amount of renal parenchyma supplied by this renal artery was too large to sacrifice using embolization.

Essential hypertension is present in many patients with and without renal artery stenosis and is in fact a much more common etiology of hypertension than renovascular disease. For this reason, renovascular hypertension can be challenging to properly diagnose. Given the end-organ consequences of uncontrolled hypertension and the potential complications of renal artery interventions, this distinction is critical to make accurately.

Several adjuncts to anatomic diagnosis can help clarify whether a renal artery intervention should be performed. Direct arterial pressure measurements at the time of angiography determine if a significant (>10 mm Hg systolic) pressure gradient is present across the stenosis. Captopril renal scintigraphy can demonstrate whether asymmetric renal perfusion is present, and it might also demonstrate the relative function of each kidney. Selective renal vein renin sampling that lateralizes to a kidney with a visualized renal artery stenosis can indicate the lesion's clinical significance.

Notes

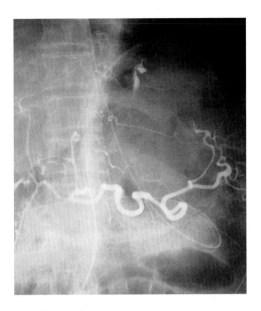 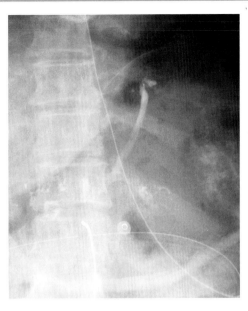

1. What is the diagnosis?

2. What artery most commonly supplies this region?

3. What embolization agent is preferred?

4. If endoscopic examination clearly visualizes a bleeding mucosal tear near the esophagogastric junction but no active extravasation is seen on angiography, what should be done?

CASE 114

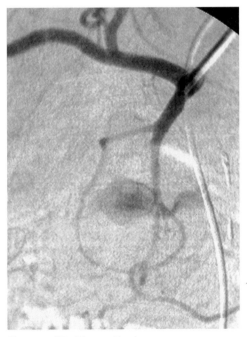 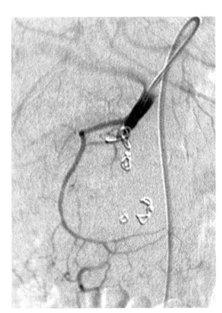

Courtesy of Dr. Thomas Vesely.   *Courtesy of Dr. Thomas Vesely.*

1. What vascular problem is pictured in the first image?

2. Name two common causes of this problem.

3. What treatment options are commonly used for this problem?

4. Is vasopressin infusion or embolization more likely to be effective?

CASE 113

Mallory–Weiss Tear

1. Mallory–Weiss tear.

2. Left gastric artery.

3. Gelfoam.

4. The left gastric artery should be embolized anyway.

Reference

Morales P, Baum AE. Therapeutic alternatives for the Mallory–Weiss tear. *Curr Treat Options Gastroenterol.* 2003;6:75-83.

Cross-Reference

Vascular and Interventional Radiology: THE REQUISITES, pp 298-304.

Comment

A Mallory–Weiss tear is the most common nonvariceal source of bleeding at the esophagogastric junction. It most commonly results from a single linear nontransmural tear on the gastric side of the junction. The typical patient is an alcoholic who has suffered repetitive emesis. Therefore, endoscopy is critical to differentiate this disorder from variceal hemorrhage, a diagnosis that is also common in this patient population.

When endoscopic intervention fails to produce cessation of bleeding, arteriography is requested. Although focal accumulations of contrast medium may be seen lining the tear or the adjacent gastric folds (occasionally producing the pseudovein sign seen in the second image above), in many cases active contrast extravasation is not identified. Because of the rich collateral supply to the stomach via the gastroepiploic arteries, short gastric arteries, and right gastric artery, the left gastric artery can be embolized whether active extravasation is seen.

CASE 114

Bleeding Duodenal Ulcer

1. Gastroduodenal artery extravasation with pseudoaneurysm formation.

2. Duodenal ulcer, pancreatitis.

3. Endoscopic therapy, surgical treatment, and percutaneous embolization.

4. Embolization.

Reference

Levkovitz Z, Cappell MS, Lookstein R, et al. Radiologic diagnosis and treatment of gastrointestinal hemorrhage and ischemia. *Med Clin North Am.* 2002;86:1357-1399.

Cross-Reference

Vascular and Interventional Radiology: THE REQUISITES, pp 298-304.

Comment

Upper gastrointestinal (GI) bleeding is typically initially evaluated and managed with endoscopy. However, when endoscopic therapy fails, angiography may be indicated. The gastroduodenal artery runs immediately behind the first part of the duodenum. Consequently, ulcers penetrating its posterior wall can cause life-threatening arterial bleeding into the GI tract.

Depending upon the endoscopically determined location of bleeding, patients with upper GI bleeding are evaluated with selective arteriography of either the celiac artery (most of the time) or superior mesenteric artery. The parent catheter or a microcatheter can then be used to subselect the bleeding artery (in this case the gastroduodenal artery). If contrast extravasation is observed, embolization is performed using either Gelfoam or coils (second image). When using coils, it is important to be sure to embolize from distal to proximal to prevent backfilling of the ulcer from the gastroepiploic system (via the splenic artery) or the pancreaticoduodenal arcade (via the superior mesenteric artery). Given the intermittent nature of GI bleeding, if contrast extravasation cannot be confirmed, embolization of the gastroduodenal artery should still be performed if the endoscopic findings were clear or if the patient is unstable. Embolization therapy, while highly effective in producing initial cessation of bleeding and in stabilizing the patient, is less likely to provide a durable solution for large ulcers, and surgical therapy might ultimately be needed.

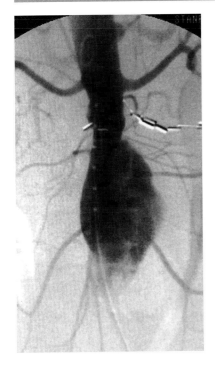
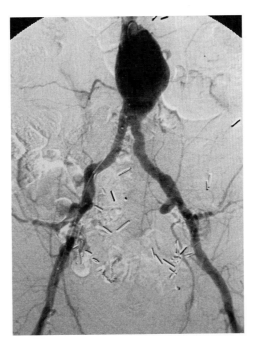
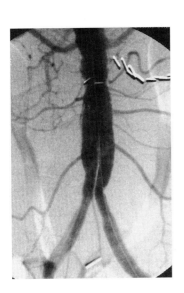
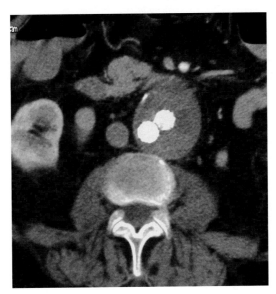

1. What procedure has been performed?

2. Is this procedure associated with less operative morbidity than open repair?

3. Name two procedure-related complications of this procedure.

4. Name three potential late complications of this procedure.

Endoluminal Graft Repair of Abdominal Aortic Aneurysm

1. Endoluminal graft repair of abdominal aortic aneurysm (AAA).

2. Yes.

3. Iliac artery rupture, branch vessel occlusion.

4. Endoleak, graft limb occlusion, device migration.

Reference

Zarins CK, White RA, Schwarten D, et al. AneuRx stent graft versus open surgical repair of abdominal aortic aneurysms: Multicenter prospective clinical trial. *J Vasc Surg.* 1999;29:292-308.

Cross-Reference

Vascular and Interventional Radiology: THE REQUI-SITES, pp 256-260.

Comment

Endovascular repair (stent-graft placement) of AAA has been increasingly used since 1991. Endovascular repair of AAA is associated with reduced hospital stay, periprocedural morbidity, and need for blood transfusions compared with open repair. By enabling treatment of patients with significant comorbidities, this procedure has expanded the range of patients who can be offered aneurysm repair. However, strict anatomic criteria must be used to select appropriate candidates for this procedure.

Advances in device technology have made it technically feasible to perform the procedure through a percutaneous approach without the need for femoral artery cutdown. Fluoroscopic guidance is used throughout the procedure. An aortogram is performed. Over a stiff wire, a large delivery sheath is carefully advanced into the aorta and, following repeat angiography, the trunk component is deployed with its upper end just below the lowest renal artery origin and expanded by angioplasty. The contralateral limb is catheterized from the other femoral artery, and repeat angiography is performed to define the distal neck of the contralateral side. The contralateral component is then deployed overlapping with the trunk component and expanded by angioplasty. Final angiography is performed to ensure that the graft limbs are patent, no endoleak is present, and all previously noted branch vessels are still patent (third image). The groins are then closed surgically if femoral cutdown was performed, or they are closed by percutaneous arterial closure devices if the procedure was performed in a completely percutaneous

manner. After the procedure, patients are followed diligently with CT angiography (final image) and abdominal x-rays to evaluate for endoleak and late endograft migration.

Notes

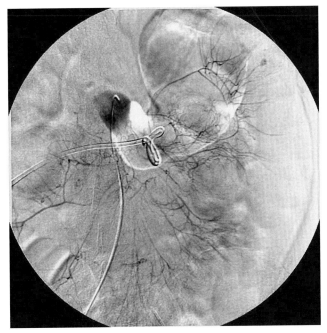

Courtesy of Dr. Michael Darcy.

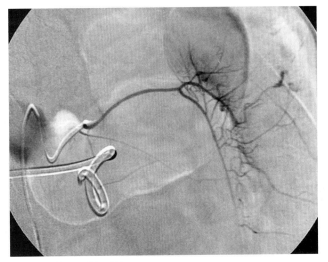

Courtesy of Dr. Michael Darcy.

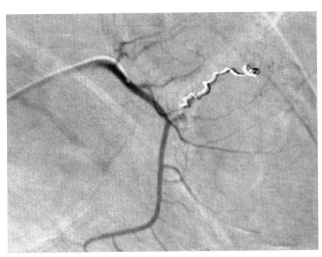

Courtesy of Dr. Michael Darcy.

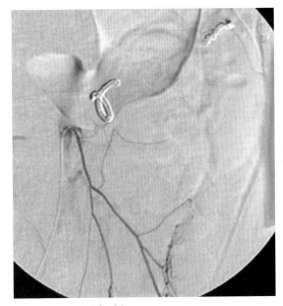

Courtesy of Dr. Michael Darcy.

1. What problem is seen in this man with lower gastrointestinal bleeding (LGIB)?

2. What mesenteric branch vessels were successively catheterized?

3. Could vasopressin infusion have been performed to treat this abnormality?

4. How often is symptomatic ischemia observed following superselective colonic artery embolization?

Embolization of Lower Gastrointestinal Bleeding

1. Focal contrast extravasation from a left colon diverticulum.

2. Superior mesenteric artery (SMA), middle colic artery, marginal artery.

3. Yes.

4. From 1% to 4% of cases.

Reference

Darcy MD. Treatment of lower gastrointestinal bleeding: Vasopressin infusion versus embolization. *J Vasc Intervent Radiol.* 2003;14:535-543.

Cross-Reference

Vascular and Interventional Radiology: THE REQUI-SITES, pp 298-304.

Comment

Contraindications to vasopressin therapy for LGIB include coronary artery and cerebrovascular disease, arrhythmia, and severe hypertension. Vasopressin infusion has largely been replaced by coil embolization for treating LGIB. The main reason underlying this change is the development of microcatheter technology, which has enabled rapid catheterization of very small arterial branches and fairly easy traversal of tortuous vascular segments. Because colonic branches are often easy to catheterize rapidly, embolotherapy can be a fast way of obtaining hemostasis. Generally, coils are used for embolization of LGIB, although a variety of materials including Gelfoam and polyvinyl alcohol particles have also been used. Since the advent of superselective embolization using microcatheters, symptomatic ischemia following embolization has been extremely uncommon.

It is very important to account for the collateral supply in the bowel when treating GI bleeding. For example, the splenic flexure is usually supplied by a marginal artery that connects the SMA and inferior mesenteric (IMA) arterial circulations (third image). For this reason, in the case presented here, coils were placed in a branch of the marginal artery distal to the point of connection between the SMA and IMA circulations. Following embolization, the SMA and IMA (final image) were injected to confirm that hemostasis was achieved.

Notes

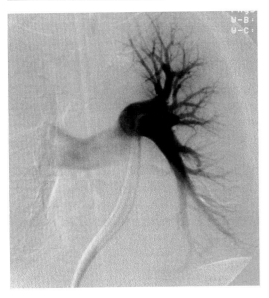
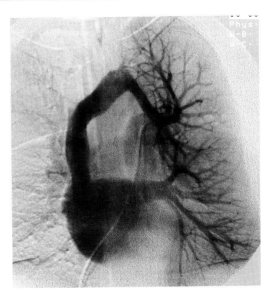

1. What vessels are opacified on the second image from this selective left pulmonary arteriogram?

2. What is the diagnosis?

3. Would this abnormality cause cyanosis?

4. Is this abnormality associated with congenital heart disease?

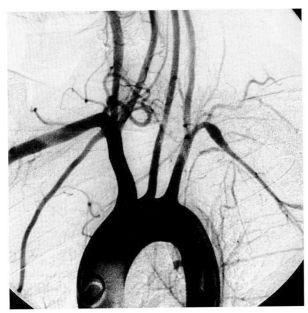
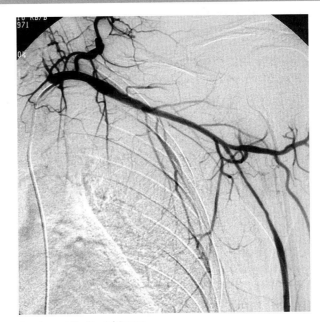

Courtesy of Dr. Daniel Brown. *Courtesy of Dr. Daniel Brown.*

1. What is the probable diagnosis in this young patient?

2. Is this disorder more common in males or females?

3. In what situations can angioplasty be performed?

4. Can the pulmonary arteries be involved with this disease?

CASE 117

Partial Anomalous Pulmonary Venous Return

1. Left upper-lobe pulmonary vein, left brachiocephalic vein, superior vena cava.

2. Partial anomalous pulmonary venous return (PAPVR).

3. No.

4. Yes.

Reference

Hong YK, Park YW, Ryu SJ, et al. Efficacy of MRI in complicated congenital heart disease with visceral heterotaxy syndrome. *J Comput Assist Tomogr.* 2000; 24:671-682.

Cross-Reference

Vascular and Interventional Radiology: THE REQUISITES, pp 194-197.

Comment

The true incidence of partial anomalous PAPVR is difficult to determine because many patients are asymptomatic. Symptoms typically arise from associated congenital heart defects or from increased pulmonary flow and right heart volume overload resulting from left-to-right shunting. Symptoms are rarely seen when less than 50% of pulmonary venous blood returns to the right atrium.

A number of congenital cardiac defects have been identified in association with PAPVR. The most common is an atrial septal defect, particularly when the PAPVR drains the right lung to the superior vena cava (SVC). Other associated cardiac defects include ventricular septal defect (VSD), tetralogy of Fallot, pulmonary valve atresia with VSD, aortic coarctation, common atrium, and single ventricle.

There are multiple forms of PAPVR, and one or several veins may be involved. The right lung is more commonly affected, and, rarely, both lungs are involved. The most common is an anomalous connection between the right upper-lobe pulmonary vein and the SVC. PAPVR from the right lower-lobe pulmonary vein to the inferior vena cava is called *scimitar syndrome* because of its classic plain film appearance.

CASE 118

Takayasu's Arteritis

1. Takayasu's arteritis.

2. Females more than males (3:1 ratio).

3. When flow-limiting stenosis is present and the patient's inflammatory disease is not in an active phase.

4. Yes.

Reference

Weyand CM, Goronzy JJ. Medium- and large-vessel vasculitis. *N Engl J Med.* 2003;349:160-169.

Cross-Reference

Vascular and Interventional Radiology: THE REQUISITES, pp 275-276.

Comment

Takayasu's arteritis is a granulomatous vasculitis that primarily involves the thoracic and abdominal aorta and its large branch vessels. Because of infiltration of the adventitia with inflammatory cells, the luminal caliber of the vessel is compromised and fibrotic stenoses eventually develop. It is more common in women younger than 50 years. Patients characteristically have an elevated erythrocyte sedimentation rate, and approximately half exhibit constitutional symptoms in the acute inflammatory stage including myalgias, fatigue, low-grade fever, tachycardia, and pain adjacent to the inflamed arteries. Interestingly, there may be a 5- to 20-year interval between the onset of acute inflammatory symptoms and the development of symptomatic arterial occlusive disease. Patients typically present with neurologic symptoms, history of stroke, or asymmetric arm blood pressure measurements and/or pulses.

Aortography typically shows smooth concentric narrowing of the aorta and/or branch vessel stenoses or occlusions. In 75% of cases the aortic arch and branch vessels are affected. The left subclavian artery is commonly affected (55%), followed in decreasing order of frequency by the right subclavian artery, left common carotid artery, and right common carotid artery. In the case presented here, there is a smooth, elongated stenosis of the left axillosubclavian artery, a fairly characteristic appearance.

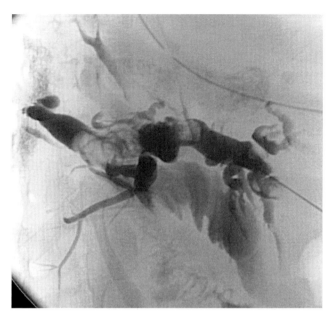

Courtesy of Dr. Daniel Brown.

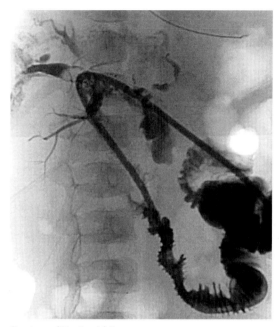

Courtesy of Dr. Daniel Brown.

1. What surgical procedure has been performed?

2. What symptoms are probably present?

3. What abnormality is seen?

4. What is the probable etiology?

Postoperative Biliary Calculi

1. Hepaticojejunostomy.

2. Right upper quadrant pain, jaundice, itching.

3. Globular filling defects within the right and left hepatic ducts.

4. Calculi or blood clots.

Reference

De Moor V, El Nakadi I, Jeanmart J, et al. Cholangitis caused by Roux-en-Y hepaticojejunostomy obstruction by a biliary stone after liver transplantation. *Transplantation*. 2003;75:416-418.

Cross-Reference

Vascular and Interventional Radiology: THE REQUISITES, pp 584-586.

Comment

The images demonstrate a surgical hepaticojejunostomy, in which the common hepatic duct was anastomosed to a loop of proximal small bowel. Several large, globular filling defects are present within the ducts, representing biliary calculi.

Patients with biliary–enteric anastomoses can develop several types of complications. The most significant early complication is anastomotic leakage. Also, early on, poor drainage of bile may be present during the first week due to edema at the biliary–enteric anastomosis.

Several potential late complications exist. The development of an anastomotic stricture can lead to episodes of cholangitis. Such strictures can be treated with prolonged biliary drainage and balloon dilation. The late complication pictured in the images here is the development of biliary calculi, which occurs in a small percentage of patients following this surgical procedure. Because the common presence of a Roux-en-Y limb can render endoscopic intervention impossible in many cases, percutaneous methods of removing or dislodging calculi are desirable in many such patients. With Roux-en-Y limbs, obstruction of the afferent loop also occurs in a small percentage of patients.

Notes

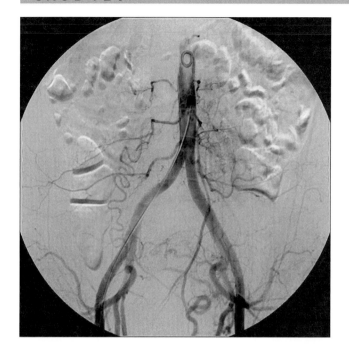
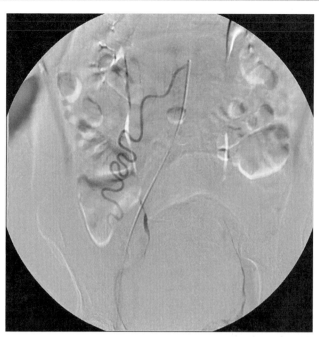
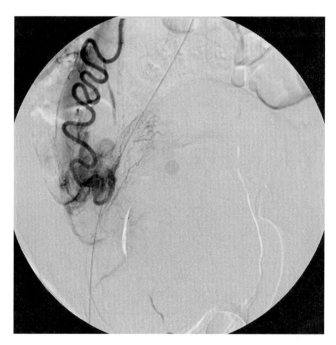

1. What percentage of patients do not exhibit clinical response following uterine fibroid embolization?

2. How is clinical success monitored after the procedure?

3. Name two potential causes of failure of uterine fibroid embolization.

4. Why did this patient fail uterine artery embolization and what can be done?

Ovarian Artery Embolization

1. About 10% to 15%.

2. Patient history (to evaluate symptoms) and MRI (to evaluate fibroid and uterus size).

3. Uterine artery spasm, aberrant arterial supply to the fibroid uterus.

4. Supply to the fibroids via the right ovarian artery. This artery was embolized, resulting in clinical treatment success.

Reference

Worthington-Kirsch RL, Andrews RT, Siskin GP, et al. Uterine fibroid embolization: Technical aspects. *Tech Vasc Intervent Radiol.* 2002;5(1):17-34.

Cross-Reference

Vascular and Interventional Radiology: THE REQUI-SITES, pp 372-373.

Comment

Uterine artery embolization has been shown to improve menorrhagia symptoms and pelvic pain in 85% to 90% of patients. There are several potential reasons why a minority of patients do not demonstrate clinical response after embolization. One potential reason is incomplete bilateral embolization. The most common reason this might occur is when arterial spasm-related slow flow in the uterine artery deceives the angiographer into believing that embolization has been achieved. Another common reason is the presence of additional blood supply to the fibroid uterus. This can result from congenital variations in uterine artery anatomy or to pelvic collateral supply.

The images here demonstrate the most common source of extrauterine supply to the uterus: an enlarged ovarian artery. In the first image, the right ovarian artery is clearly visualized on the nonselective aortic injection, confirming that it is abnormally enlarged. The final two images demonstrate the characteristic serpiginous appearance of the ovarian artery and its eventual supply to the right part of the uterine fundus.

Fortunately, the ovarian artery can also be embolized. Most interventionalists embolize the main ovarian artery using Gelfoam, although some advance a microcatheter beyond the ovary and attempt subselective embolization of the uterine branches.

Notes

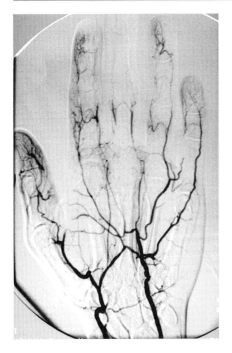
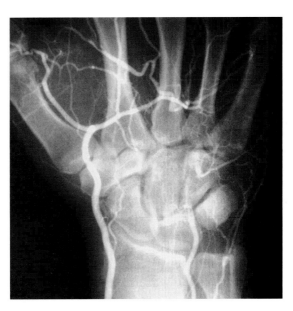

1. Which vessel is abnormal in these two patients?

2. What is the anatomic reason for this vessel's vulnerability?

3. What anatomic factor is an important determinant of symptom severity?

4. Does this abnormality tend to produce distal embolization?

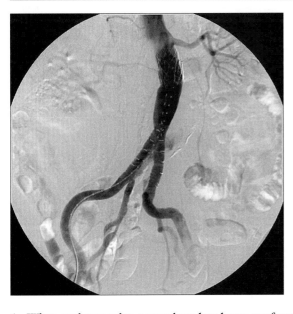
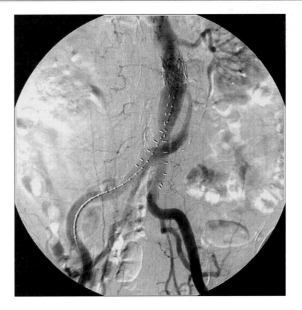

1. What endovascular procedure has been performed?

2. How are patients usually monitored following this procedure?

3. What abnormality is present on this angiogram?

4. Why is this significant?

Hypothenar Hammer Syndrome

1. Ulnar artery.

2. It can be compressed against the hook of the hamate.

3. The degree of completeness of the palmar arch.

4. Yes (see the first image above).

Reference

Anderson SE, De Monaco D, Buechler U, et al. Imaging features of pseudoaneurysms of the hand in children and adults. *Am J Roentgenol.* 2003;180:659-664.

Cross-Reference

Vascular and Interventional Radiology: THE REQUI-SITES, pp 159-160.

Comment

Hypothenar hammer syndrome is an uncommon cause of digital ischemia that occurs as a result of repetitive blunt trauma or mechanical vibration or pressure to the wrist or palm. Typically it is the result of occupational trauma (e.g., jackhammer operators), and it can be seen in persons who practice martial arts. Lesser forms of trauma, including repetitive microtrauma in typists or pianists, can also lead to digital ischemia.

The chronic trauma produces spasm and intimal injury resulting in thrombosis (second image) and/or formation of a pseudoaneurysm (first image). A pseudoaneurysm might serve as a source of emboli to the digital arteries (first image). Although other vessels can be affected, the ulnar artery is particularly vulnerable where it crosses the hamate bone and can be compressed.

The degree of symptomatology depends upon vessel patency, the presence of emboli, and the degree of completeness of the palmar arch. Symptoms include evidence of digital ischemia, Raynaud's phenomenon, and/or a pulsatile mass.

Type I Endoleak

1. Endoluminal graft insertion.

2. Periodic cross-sectional imaging with CT angiography using noncontrast, arterial phase contrast-enhanced, and delayed postcontrast imaging.

3. Type I endoleak from the right distal attachment site.

4. Potential for aneurysm rupture.

Reference

Tummala S, Powell A. Imaging of endoleaks. *Tech Vasc Intervent Radiol.* 2001;4(4):208-212.

Cross-Reference

Vascular and Interventional Radiology: THE REQUI-SITES, pp 256-260.

Comment

An endoleak is defined as the persistence of blood flow outside the graft within the aneurysm sac following endoluminal repair. An aneurysm sac that is completely excluded from flow typically thromboses and often shrinks in diameter. The presence of perigraft flow leaves the aneurysm at risk for enlargement and/or rupture. The images here clearly depict a type I leak, with filling of the aneurysm sac on the second image.

Endoleaks are classified by type. Type I endoleaks result from flow around the ends of the endograft and are subdivided into type IA (proximal attachment site leak) and IB (distal attachment site leak). These endoleaks require urgent therapy. Type II endoleaks are the most common and result from retrograde arterial flow into the aneurysm sac from patent aortic side-branches (typically lumbar, sacral, gonadal, accessory renal, or inferior mesenteric artery branches). The criteria upon which to base treatment of type II endoleaks are controversial. Some physicians treat all type II leaks via side-branch embolization or glue embolization of the aneurysm sac, and others believe that watchful waiting is sufficient provided the aneurysm is not enlarging. Type III endoleaks are rare and result from tears in the graft fabric or separation of graft components. Type IV endoleaks represent leakage of contrast due to porosity of the graft fabric material.

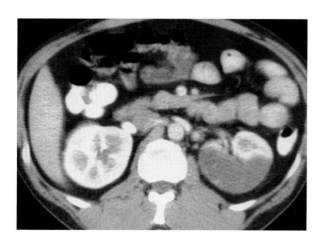
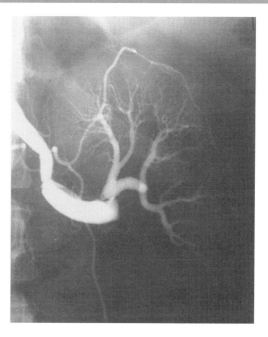

1. What abnormality is seen on the CT scan of this young woman with acute left flank pain?

2. What is the cause of this patient's pain?

3. What is the most common cause of this problem when it occurs spontaneously?

4. What is the most common overall cause of this problem?

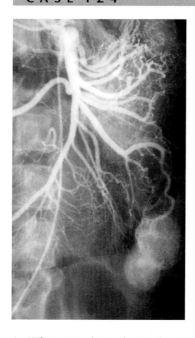

1. What vessel is selectively opacified?

2. What abnormality is present?

3. Where is this abnormality most likely located?

4. What is the most likely reason this angiogram was performed?

CASE 123

Spontaneous Renal Artery Dissection

1. Severe hypoperfusion of the posterior part of the left kidney.

2. Left renal artery dissection.

3. Fibromuscular dysplasia.

4. Iatrogenic renal artery injury during angioplasty.

Reference

Muller BT, Reiher L, Pfeiffer T, et al. Surgical treatment of renal artery dissection in 25 patients: Indications and results. *J Vasc Surg.* 2003;37:761-768.

Cross-Reference

Vascular and Interventional Radiology: THE REQUISITES, pp 327-336.

Comment

The second image demonstrates apparent enlargement and double-density of the left renal artery with a proximal focal indentation consistent with a renal artery dissection. The flap extends to the bifurcation of the main left renal artery, and its posterior division is occluded. This explains the marked left kidney hypoperfusion on CT.

Renal artery aneurysm and/or renal artery dissection occur in a minority of patients with fibromuscular dysplasia. Given the rarity of other etiologies of these lesions, however, a patient with an unexplained renal artery aneurysm or dissection is highly likely to have underlying fibromuscular dysplasia.

Patients with spontaneous renal artery dissection are nearly always managed with surgical aortorenal arterial bypass. In patients who are poor candidates for surgery, stents can be used to treat focal dissections limited to the main renal artery.

CASE 124

Small Bowel Leiomyoma

1. Superior mesenteric artery.

2. A well-circumscribed, bilobed enhancing mass.

3. Small bowel.

4. Evaluation of chronic lower gastrointestinal bleeding.

Reference

Lefkovitz Z, Cappel MS, Kaplan M, et al. Radiology in the diagnosis and therapy of gastrointestinal bleeding. *Gastroenterol Clin North Am.* 2000;29:489-512.

Cross-Reference

Vascular and Interventional Radiology: THE REQUISITES, p 304.

Comment

Many patients develop chronic GI blood loss but have negative workups, including upper and lower endoscopies, small bowel follow-through, and tagged RBC scintigraphy. In such cases, angiography can sometimes help to identify an occult vascular lesion such as angiodysplasia or a small bowel tumor, with the goal of providing guidance for surgical resection. Owing to the intermittent low-grade bleeding associated with these lesions, extravasation of contrast is not typically seen during angiography.

Although small bowel tumors are rarely seen at arteriography, an understanding of their basic imaging features is useful to have. Leiomyomas like the one depicted here have a characteristic appearance with well-circumscribed margins, prominent feeding arteries and draining veins, and irregular corkscrew tumor vessels with a dense tumor stain. Most are benign, although malignancy cannot be excluded on imaging. The most common primary tumor of small bowel is carcinoid. Owing to its prominent desmoplastic reaction within the mesentery, characteristic angiographic findings include retraction, displacement, and occlusions of multiple superior mesenteric artery branches. Hamartomas and adenocarcinomas typically appear hypovascular. Lymphomas have no characteristic findings. They can demonstrate vascular displacement or encasement but are often undetectable despite widespread involvement.

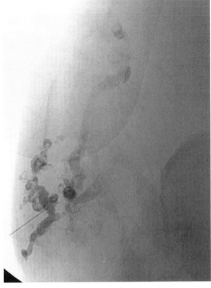

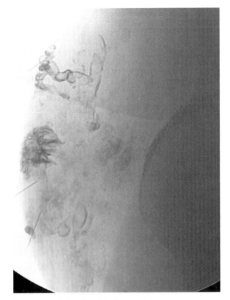

Courtesy of Dr. David Hovsepian.　　　　*Courtesy of Dr. David Hovsepian.*

1. Why might this patient have presented for evaluation and treatment?

2. What is the most likely diagnosis?

3. What is the first-line imaging method of choice for these lesions?

4. How can this be treated percutaneously?

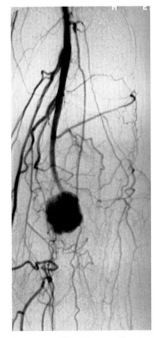

Courtesy of Dr. Thomas Vesely.

1. What findings are present on this magnified arteriogram at the knee level?

2. What is the most likely cause based solely upon the angiographic findings?

3. What might this lesion represent if the patient is an intravenous drug abuser?

4. What symptoms might be present if that was the case?

ANSWERS

CASE 125

Venous Malformation

1. Local pain and swelling; in this 21-year-old police officer, his gunbelt was very uncomfortable.

2. Venous malformation.

3. Magnetic resonance imaging.

4. Direct injection of a sclerosant such as 100% ethanol.

Reference

Lee BB, Do YS, Byun HS, et al. Advanced management of venous malformation with ethanol sclerotherapy: Mid-term results. *J Vasc Surg.* 2003;37:533-538.

Cross-Reference

Vascular and Interventional Radiology: THE REQUISITES, pp 466-467.

Comment

Vascular malformations are congenital lesions that grow periodically, often in relation to trauma, surgery, or hormonal stimulation (via puberty, pregnancy, or hormonal therapy). Vascular malformations are typically categorized into arterial, capillary, venous, lymphatic, and mixed subtypes. MRI is useful to determine the depth and extent of these lesions as well as their proximity to normal structures. MRI is also useful in the imaging follow-up after treatment because multiple ablation sessions are often necessary.

Owing to the presence of an intervening capillary network, the inflow arteries to venous malformations, like the one depicted, are normal in size. Flow within these dilated abnormal veins tends to be slow or stagnant, and calcified phleboliths may be identified.

Small, asymptomatic venous malformations in the extremities are treated conservatively with compressive stockings and follow-up. Surgical resection is not indicated owing to the difficulty in extricating these delicate vascular structures from surrounding normal tissues. Sclerotherapy is favored, and absolute ethanol is the agent preferred by many. After the lesion is directly punctured with a needle, contrast is injected to confirm needle placement and determine the volume necessary to fill the lesion. A similar volume of ethanol is then injected and allowed to dwell in the lesion for about 10 minutes. Follow-up venography is performed to confirm thrombosis of the lesion.

CASE 126

Mycotic Aneurysm

1. Irregular distal popliteal artery aneurysm with occlusion of the tibial arteries.

2. Post-traumatic pseudoaneurysm.

3. Mycotic aneurysm.

4. Fever, local tenderness, positive blood cultures, and/or expanding mass.

Reference

Patra P, Ricco J, Costargent A, et al. Infected aneurysms of neck and limb arteries: A retrospective multicenter study. *Ann Vasc Surg.* 2001;15:197-205.

Cross-Reference

Vascular and Interventional Radiology: THE REQUISITES, pp 435-436.

Comment

Infectious (mycotic) aneurysms can occur anywhere in the arterial system. The usual cultured infectious organisms are *Salmonella, Streptococcus,* or *Staphylococcus* species, and the latter is commonly found in intravenous drug abusers.

Mycotic aneurysms represent an infection of the artery wall itself either caused by seeding of a preexisting aneurysm or by primary infection of a normal artery with subsequent dilation. The infection can be introduced from infected blood in the lumen or vasa vasorum, by spread from a neighboring soft tissue infection, or from penetrating trauma. Therefore, mycotic aneurysms can be true or false aneurysms and may be single or multiple depending upon the underlying condition of the vessel and the method of infection. The symptomatology and angiographic appearance can differentiate these from degenerative aneurysms. The mycotic aneurysm sac is typically irregular, saccular, and eccentric, and the arterial system is less likely to show chronic atherosclerosis.

Treatment consists of antibiotics, surgical resection of the aneurysm, débridement of infected tissues, and drainage of the infected region. In some cases the artery can be ligated, but when revascularization is necessary, an extra-anatomic bypass can often be performed to avoid the infected region. In some cases, an anatomic bypass can successfully be performed with autogenous materials (native veins) or cryopreserved allografts if success in clearing of infection with antimicrobial agents is anticipated. Prosthetic material should not be inserted into a known infected space.

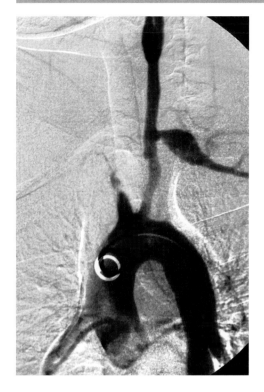

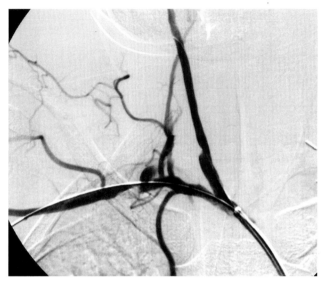

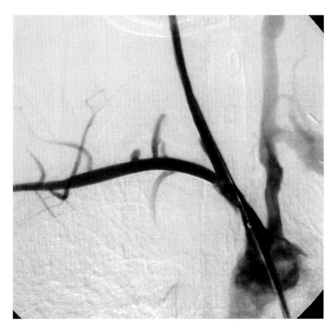

1. What is the underlying diagnosis?

2. What procedure has been performed in the second and third images?

3. Is this the first-line treatment for this problem?

4. What is the expected 5-year patency of surgical carotid–subclavian bypass in patients with atherosclerosis?

Brachiocephalic Artery Stent Placement

1. Takayasu's arteritis.

2. Stent placement in the innominate, right common carotid, and right subclavian arteries.

3. No. Carotid–subclavian bypass is the first-line treatment.

4. More than 95%.

Reference

Sharma BK, Jain S, Bali HK, et al. A follow-up study of balloon angioplasty and de-novo stenting in Takayasu arteritis. *Int J Cardiol.* 2000;75(Suppl):S147-S152.

Cross-Reference

Vascular and Interventional Radiology: THE REQUI-SITES, pp 149-151.

Comment

Patients with Takayasu's arteritis can present complex management problems. Typically they are first managed with anti-inflammatory therapy until arterial symptoms develop. At this point, surgical bypass is the usual therapy employed, although angioplasty and/or stent placement can also be used for focal, short-segment lesions that are in a chronic phase. Surgery or interventional therapy in the acute inflammatory stages should be avoided owing to lower rates of long-term success.

If the brachiocephalic artery or proximal subclavian artery is occluded and the ipsilateral common carotid artery is normal, reimplantation of the subclavian artery into the carotid or carotid–subclavian bypass is the preferred operation. If the carotid artery is diseased, it is replaced with graft material, and the subclavian artery is implanted into the graft or grafted to the aorta or carotid graft.

In the case presented here, the patient had been operated on multiple times for the brachiocephalic artery occlusion and had multiple occluded bypass grafts. Because she was thought to be a poor risk for further intervention in the same operative bed, an endovascular stent was placed.

Notes

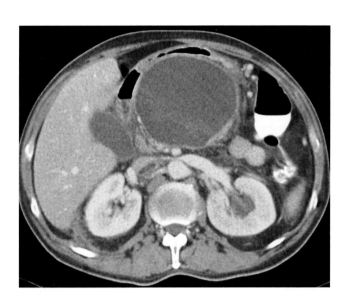 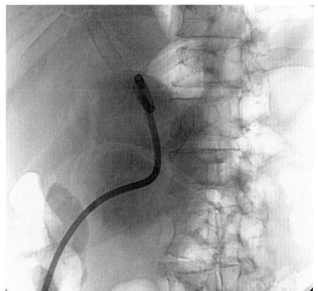

1. This patient presented with constant abdominal pain 6 weeks after an episode of acute pancreatitis. What is the diagnosis?

2. Do all patients with this diagnosis need interventional treatment?

3. What approaches can be used for draining these lesions?

4. Will this tube be ready to remove within 2 weeks?

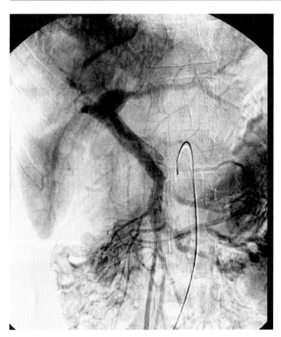

1. What procedure was performed?

2. What abnormality is present?

3. Could a celiac arteriogram diagnose this abnormality?

4. Can the underlying problem in this patient be treated with embolization therapy?

C A S E 1 2 8

Transgastric Pancreatic Pseudocyst Drainage

1. Pancreatic pseudocyst.

2. No.

3. Percutaneous transabdominal if a suitable window is present, percutaneous transgastric, endoscopic internal drainage, surgical drainage.

4. No. Pseudocyst drains are often in for months.

Reference

Neff R. Pancreatic pseudocysts and fluid collections: Percutaneous approaches. *Surg Clin North Am.* 2001; 81:399-403.

Cross-Reference

Vascular and Interventional Radiology: THE REQUISITES, pp 502-506.

Comment

Patients with fluid collections that appear after an episode of acute pancreatitis are typically initially treated with supportive care and observation. The two primary clinical situations in which pseudocyst drainage is indicated are when there is reason to suspect that a particular fluid collection is infected and when the patient has persistent pain at least 6 weeks following the initial pancreatitis episode.

The CT scan shown here demonstrates a large pancreatic pseudocyst immediately posterior to the stomach. A suitable window directly into this collection could not be identified, so transgastric drainage was performed. Given the large size of this pseudocyst, the procedure was performed using fluoroscopic guidance alone, using the indentation upon the gastric air pattern as a landmark for the location of the pseudocyst. Because pancreatic collections typically contain semisolid debris, a large-bore catheter was placed. Because transgastric pseudocyst drainage catheters are prone to displacement back into the stomach due to gastric peristalsis, a locking loop catheter was used.

Pancreatic pseudocysts typically require several months of drainage before they can be removed. In general, the criteria for removing the catheter include minimal output (<10 mL/day for 2 days), absence of fistula to the pancreatic duct, and good clinical status (the patient is afebrile and generally improved).

C A S E 1 2 9

Right Portal Vein Obstruction

1. Superior mesenteric arteriogram.

2. Right portal vein obstruction.

3. Yes.

4. No. Hepatic arterial chemoembolization would be risky owing to the presence of right portal vein occlusion: Hepatic ischemia might result.

Reference

Uflacker R. Applications of percutaneous mechanical thrombectomy in transjugular intrahepatic portosystemic shunt and portal vein thrombosis. *Tech Vasc Interv Radiol.* 2003;6(1):59-69.

Cross-Reference

Vascular and Interventional Radiology: THE REQUISITES, p 402.

Comment

It is always important to evaluate the arterial, parenchymal, and venous phases of any arteriogram. The image here represents the venous phase of a superior mesenteric arteriogram. The superior mesenteric vein, main portal vein, and left portal vein are clearly patent. There is occlusion of the right portal vein, which in this patient was due to malignancy. The angiogram was being performed to evaluate the feasibility of chemoembolization therapy for this patient's hepatocellular carcinoma.

Portal vein thrombosis can be caused by primary hepatic or metastatic tumor, dehydration, sepsis, transplantation, and other hypercoagulable states. Its presence is important to the interventionalist in several clinical situations, including patients with cancer in whom hepatic chemoembolization is planned. The presence of portal vein obstruction would render such patients susceptible to developing severe hepatic ischemia were the hepatic artery to be embolized. Portal vein thrombosis is also important in patients with portal hypertension in whom transjugular intrahepatic portosystemic shunt (TIPS) is planned. In these patients, the presence of portal vein thrombosis would render portal vein access more difficult to obtain. However, TIPS can still be performed, either by accessing the left portal system or by recanalizing the occluded segment of the portal vein.

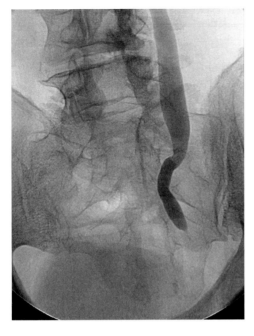 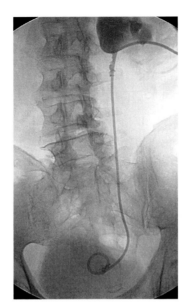

1. Name four benign causes of ureteral stricture.

2. Can benign ureteral strictures be balloon dilated with success?

3. How often does a ureteral stent need to be replaced?

4. In what patients are double-J ureteral stents relatively contraindicated?

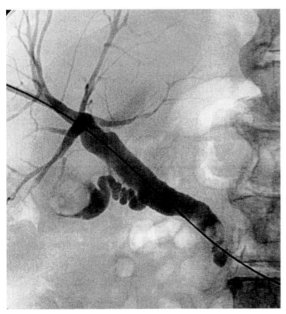

Courtesy of Dr. Daniel Brown.

1. What is the diagnosis?

2. What is the first-choice treatment in most cases?

3. What percutaneous methods can be used to treat this problem?

4. If this patient has a fever, does this need to be treated urgently?

CASE 130

Benign Ureteral Stricture

1. Scarring after ureteral calculus, after radiation therapy, iatrogenic injury during surgery, anastomosis following ileal loop diversion.

2. Yes, but the results are usually not durable.

3. Every 2 to 3 months.

4. Patients with incontinence or otherwise poor bladder function, those with urinary fistulas, those who experience refractory bladder spasms following ureteral stent placement, those who are prone to stent obstruction.

Reference

DiMarco DS, LeRoy AJ, Thieling S, et al. Long-term results of treatment for ureteroenteric strictures. *Urology*. 2001;58:909-913.

Cross-Reference

Vascular and Interventional Radiology: THE REQUISITES, pp 620-631.

Comment

These images demonstrate a tight stricture of the left ureter at the ureterovesical junction, with consequent hydroureteronephrosis. In this patient, the stricture was due to prior radiation therapy. The benign nature of this stricture is favored by its focal, smooth appearance without evidence of mass effect. That said, the radiographic appearance is fairly nonspecific, and malignancy cannot be excluded on this basis alone. The stricture was successfully crossed, and a nephroureteral stent was placed (second image).

Balloon dilation of the ureter can be effective in treating benign strictures but is associated with high recurrence rates. Recently, cutting balloons have been introduced and are used from a ureteroscopic approach with greater success. Following intervention, a stent is typically left across the stenosis to provide a scaffold for healing while preventing collapse to an unacceptable diameter.

CASE 131

Choledocholithiasis

1. Choledocholithiasis.

2. Endoscopic retrograde cholangiopancreatography (ERCP) with sphincterotomy and stone removal.

3. Balloon sphincterotomy with propulsion of the calculus into the bowel, or the calculus can be removed by a variety of grasping devices.

4. Yes.

Reference

Taylor AC, Little AF, Hennessy OF, et al. Prospective assessment of magnetic resonance cholangiopancreatography for noninvasive imaging of the biliary tree. *Gastrointest Endosc.* 2002;55(1):17-22.

Cross-Reference

Vascular and Interventional Radiology: THE REQUISITES, pp 584-586.

Comment

The image demonstrates a large filling defect within the gallbladder, consistent with calculi and/or sludge (or, less likely, tumor). The cystic duct is patent. An ovoid filling defect is present within the distal common bile duct, consistent with calculus.

Patients with choledocholithiasis can present with acute severe symptomatology (due to impaction of a mid-sized or large calculus within the common bile duct) or with chronic intermittent symptoms (due to passage of small calculi through the duct). Patients with symptoms suggesting the presence of cholangitis must be treated urgently with either stone removal or biliary drainage to rapidly relieve the obstruction. Afebrile patients with acute symptoms are usually managed with ERCP as the first-choice option. If this fails, then the patient may be referred for percutaneous biliary drainage and percutaneous stone extraction.

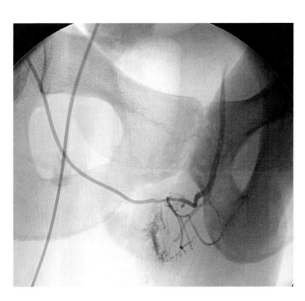
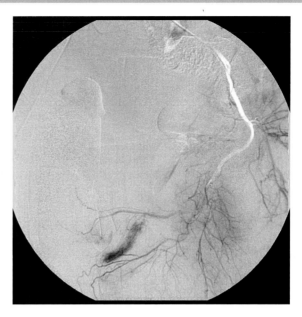

1. What diagnosis would you suspect in this patient with painful, persistent priapism following perineal trauma?

2. What pelvic artery supplies the penis?

3. What vessel is commonly injured in these patients?

4. Can this be treated using endovascular methods?

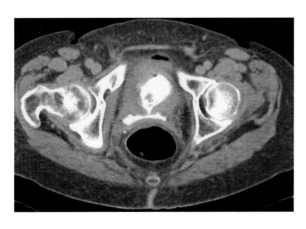
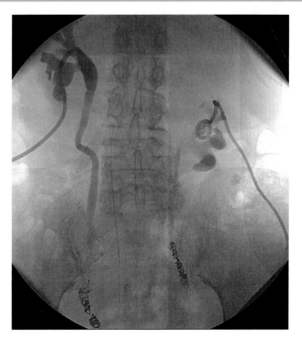

1. What is the abnormality seen on the CT cystogram in the first image?

2. What procedure has been performed in the second image?

3. Is this a temporary or permanent measure?

4. What are the indications for performing this procedure?

C A S E 1 3 2

High-Flow Priapism

1. High-flow priapism.

2. Internal pudendal artery.

3. Cavernous artery.

4. Yes, by selective embolization.

Reference

Ciampalini S, Savoca G, Buttazzi L, et al. High-flow priapism: Treatment and long-term follow-up. *Urology.* 2002;59:110-113.

Cross-Reference

Vascular and Interventional Radiology: THE REQUISITES, pp 282-283.

Comment

High-flow priapism is a rare arterial abnormality that results from direct trauma to the perineum or penis. Laceration of the cavernous artery results in development of an angiographically visible arteriolacunar fistula (first image) with direct, constant entry of arterial blood into the vascular lacuna of the erectile tissue. It helps to be familiar with the normal minor arterial blush at the base of the corpus cavernosum to be able to clearly distinguish this normal finding from the more-robust enhancement associated with a true arteriolacunar fistula (second image).

The most commonly used treatment is percutaneous embolization of the distal internal pudendal artery. Autologous blood clot and Gelfoam, both temporary agents, have been used most extensively but have a significant rate of recurrence due to subsequent recanalization. Permanent agents, such as microcoils and bucrylate glue, have also been used. Surgical ligation of the cavernous artery is also an effective treatment, but because it produces permanent occlusion it can have damaging effects on the underlying tissues.

The feared complication of both treatment and failure to treat is the development of impotence. Although many patients report a long history of high-flow priapism with normal sexual function, long-standing persistent priapism has been reported to result in fibrosis with associated erectile dysfunction. Because it is difficult to determine which patients will develop fibrosis and impotence, the timing of intervention remains controversial.

C A S E 1 3 3

Vaginovesical Fistula

1. Vaginovesical fistula.

2. Bilateral transrenal ureteral occlusion.

3. Permanent.

4. Lower urinary tract fistulas, urinary incontinence, and intractable cystitis.

Reference

Farrell TA, Wallace M, Hicks ME. Long-term results of transrenal ureteral occlusion with use of Gianturco coils and gelatin sponge pledgets. *J Vasc Interv Radiol.* 1997;8:449-452.

Cross-Reference

Vascular and Interventional Radiology: THE REQUISITES, p 629.

Comment

Lower urinary tract fistulas are abnormal communications between the urinary bladder or the distal ureters with adjacent structures (vagina, rectum, sigmoid colon, and perineum). They can develop as the result of trauma, pelvic malignancy, and radiation. Incontinence of urine is the most common presentation and has a significant impact on quality of life. Surgical repair has a high failure rate of 35% in fistulas caused by trauma and an even higher rate in those related to malignancy. Surgical diversion with ileal loop formation has been performed in such cases; however, this might not be feasible in some patients owing to poor general health or local contraindications such as pelvic malignancy or prior radiation.

Percutaneous nephrostomy drainage may be successful in allowing small fistulas to heal. Large fistulas can be managed by ureteral occlusion with permanent external urinary drainage through nephrostomy drains. A number of embolic materials have been used with varying success rates. A combination of coil and Gelfoam has been shown to have favorable technical and clinical efficacy.

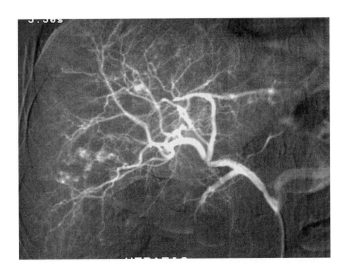

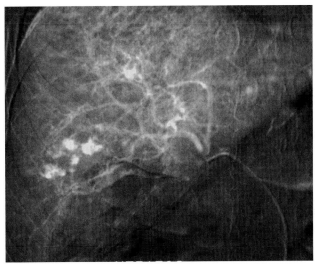

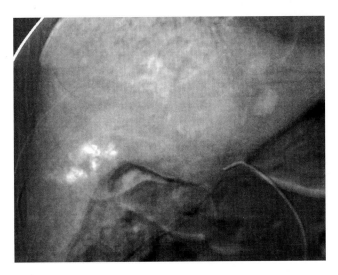

1. Which hepatic tumors demonstrate contrast pooling?

2. Which hepatic tumors demonstrate neovascularity?

3. Which hepatic tumors commonly exhibit arteriovenous shunting?

4. Which hepatic tumor is most likely in this case?

Cavernous Hemangioma of the Liver

1. Hemangioma, hepatocellular carcinoma, hepatoblastoma, angiosarcoma, and hypervascular metastases.

2. Adenoma, hepatocellular carcinoma, hepatoblastoma, cholangiocarcinoma, metastases, and occasionally focal nodular hyperplasia.

3. Hepatocellular carcinoma and giant hemangioma of infancy or hemangioendothelioma.

4. Hemangioma.

Reference

Giavraglou C, Economou H, Oannidis I. Arterial embolization of giant hepatic hemangiomas. *Cardiovasc Intervent Radiol*. 2003;26:92-96.

Cross-Reference

Vascular and Interventional Radiology: THE REQUISITES, pp 308-310.

Comment

Hemangiomas are the most common benign hepatic tumors and are typically found incidentally during cross-sectional imaging. Pathologically, they comprise endothelium-lined vascular spaces divided by thin septations and suspended in a loose fibroblastic stroma. They typically remain stable in size over time, but occasionally they grow quite large. When a hemangioma is present, symptoms are commonly related to the neoplasm size, but they rarely are due to rupture or platelet sequestration.

The arteriographic appearance is characteristic. The feeding vessels are typically normal in size unless the lesion is very large. Dense nodular opacification of the lesion starts at the periphery (first image) and progresses inward (later images). The lesions are well circumscribed and have dilated, irregular, nodule-like vascular spaces. Contrast opacification persisting well into the venous phase differentiates this lesion from other hepatic neoplasms except for the rare angiosarcoma that can mimic a hemangioma.

Other hepatic lesions that exhibit vascular pooling tend to be malignant tumors, including hepatocellular carcinoma and metastases. Similar to cross-sectional imaging characteristics, these can typically be differentiated by the shorter period of pooling, less-uniform enhancement, enlargement of the feeding artery, and neovascularity.

Notes

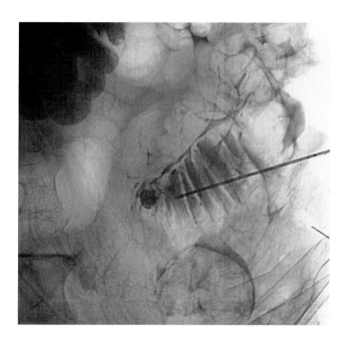

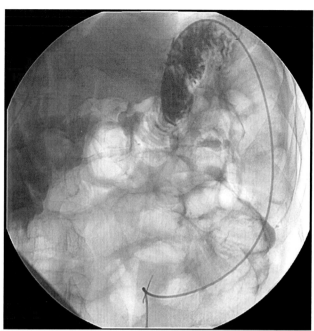

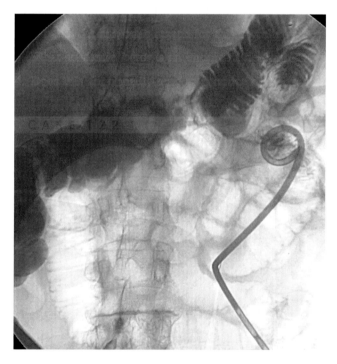

1. What procedure has been performed?

2. Name one early and one late potential complication of this procedure.

3. Can this be performed through a prior surgical jejunostomy tract?

4. What alternative methods of providing enteral nutrition are considered preferential options for most patients?

C A S E 1 3 5

Direct Percutaneous Jejunostomy

1. Direct percutaneous jejunostomy.

2. Early: peritonitis; Late: catheter occlusion.

3. Yes.

4. Surgical jejunostomy and percutaneous gastrojejunostomy.

Reference

Cope C, Davis AG, Baum RA, et al. Direct percutaneous jejunostomy: Techniques and applications—ten years experience. *Radiology*. 1998;209:747-754.

Cross-Reference

Vascular and Interventional Radiology: THE REQUI-SITES, pp 536-537.

Comment

The examination demonstrates percutaneous transabdominal placement of a jejunostomy catheter. Although surgical jejunostomy and percutaneous gastrojejunostomy represent the standard approaches for obtaining the ability to feed into the jejunum, there are occasional clinical situations in which these procedures are not possible. One common scenario is the patient who has undergone gastrectomy, esophagogastrectomy, or esophagectomy with gastric pullthrough, and who is also a poor operative risk.

Because the small bowel is usually not fixed within the abdomen and can be quite mobile, direct percutaneous jejunostomy can be technically challenging to perform. Factors that help the interventionalist include: (1) The presence of an identifiable scar from a prior surgical jejunostomy, because it is likely that the adjacent loop of small bowel has been surgically tethered to the anterior abdominal wall, making it less likely to fall away during the procedure; (2) The ability to identify a suitable loop of bowel using ultrasound guidance or using fluoroscopic examination with or without injection of air through a nasogastric catheter. Although techniques vary, many interventionalists first place a T-tack (second image) into the jejunal loop under fluoroscopic guidance and use this to maintain gentle traction on the bowel while the tract is dilated to accommodate the jejunostomy catheter. As with gastrojejunostomy, tube feedings into the small bowel are given continuously rather than in bolus fashion.

Notes

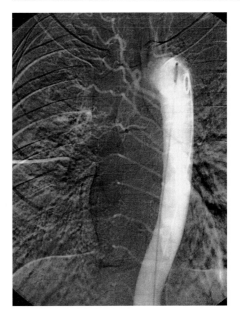
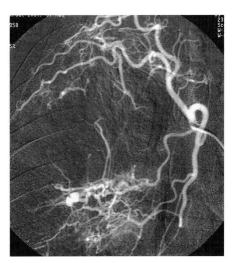

1. What artery has been selected in the second image above?

2. What procedure is normally performed before the procedure shown above?

3. What is the underlying etiology of symptoms in this patient?

4. What is a Rasmussen's aneurysm?

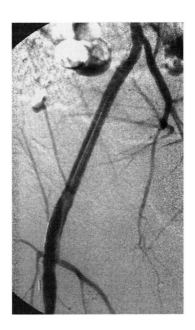
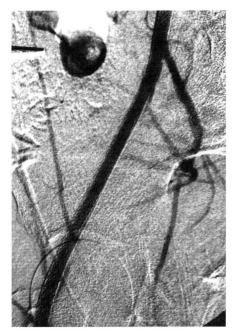

1. What abnormal finding is present on the first image above?

2. What procedure did this patient have recently that might have caused this?

3. What percutaneous method of treatment is shown in the second image?

4. Is it advisable to extend stents into the common femoral artery?

CASE 136

Cavitary Right Lung Mass

1. Right bronchial artery.

2. Bronchoscopy.

3. Cavitary right lung mass.

4. A pulmonary artery branch aneurysm due to tuberculosis.

Reference

Barben J, Robertson D, Olinsky A, et al. Bronchial artery embolization for hemoptysis in young patients with cystic fibrosis. *Radiology.* 2002;224:124-130.

Cross-Reference

Vascular and Interventional Radiology: THE REQUI-SITES, pp 215-217.

Comment

The images demonstrate a selective right bronchial arteriogram. The right bronchial arterial branches are markedly splayed, demonstrating a right upper lung mass that is hypervascular at its periphery and avascular in its central region (suggesting necrosis). The differential diagnosis includes primary lung carcinoma (which was the case in the patient shown), metastatic disease, and infectious lesions such as tuberculosis and fungal disease. In this patient, a focus of contrast extravasation was observed at the inferior margin of the lesion, presumably the source of hemoptysis. This stands in contrast to the vast majority of bronchial arteriograms for hemoptysis, in which contrast extravasation is not visualized. In this patient, palliative treatment was performed using embolization with polyvinyl alcohol particles, with subsequent cessation of bleeding.

Common reasons for severe hemoptysis include cystic fibrosis, chronic obstructive pulmonary disease, bronchiectasis, and vascular tumors such as the one depicted above.

Bronchoscopy is routinely performed before arteriographic evaluation of hemoptysis, in order to determine which bronchial segment contains the bleeding source. This greatly helps the angiographer, because many patients have enlarged bronchial arteries bilaterally with no evidence of contrast extravasation. The angiographer can then direct therapy to the artery thought likely to be causing the bleeding based upon bronchoscopy.

CASE 137

Stenting of Iliac Artery Dissection

1. A dissection flap in the right external iliac artery.

2. Stent insertion into the distal right external iliac artery.

3. Insertion of an additional stent to tack the flap down.

4. No. Stents should not be placed in areas of joint flexion when possible.

Reference

Funovics MA, Lackner B, Cejna M, et al. Predictors of long-term results after treatment of iliac artery obliteration by transluminal angioplasty and stent deployment. *Cardiovasc Intervent Radiol.* 2002;25:397-402.

Cross-Reference

Vascular and Interventional Radiology: THE REQUI-SITES, pp 270-273.

Comment

Stent placement has become an accepted method of treating a variety of arterial vascular abnormalities, including flow-limiting dissections, short-segment arterial occlusions, arterial stenoses refractory to angioplasty, arterial stenoses that recur following successful angioplasty, and eccentric or extremely calcified atherosclerotic lesions. Currently available vascular stents fall into two main categories.

Balloon-expandable stents (prototype: Palmaz stent) are generally less than 4 cm long and are premounted on an angioplasty balloon. Their primary advantage is the pinpoint accuracy with which they can be positioned, because the deployment step simply involves inflating the carrier balloon. Their primary disadvantages are the inability to treat longer lesions with a single stent and the possibility of the stent's slipping off the balloon during introduction. The latter problem has been largely remedied by stents that are securely mounted upon their carrier balloons by the manufacturer.

Self-expandable stents (prototype: Wallstent) are available in longer lengths, possess greater longitudinal flexibility, and do not require balloon mounting. However, because deployment requires a carefully controlled unsheathing of the restrained stent, allowing it to expand, these stents are slightly more prone to malpositioning during deployment.

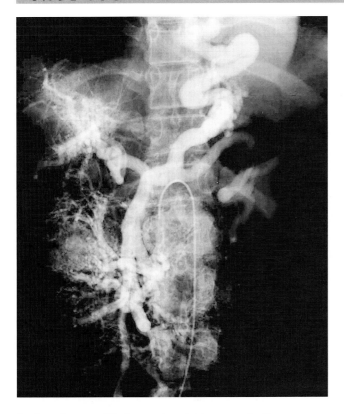

1. Are the opacified vessels arteries or veins?

2. What abnormal findings are present?

3. Are these acute or chronic findings?

4. Would wedged hepatic venography yield accurate estimates of portal pressures?

CASE 138

Cavernous Transformation of the Portal Vein

1. Veins.

2. Cavernous transformation of the portal vein and a large gastroesophageal varix.

3. Chronic.

4. No.

Reference

Gallego C, Velasco M, Marcuello P, et al. Congenital and acquired anomalies of the portal venous system. *Radiographics.* 2002;22(1):141-159.

Cross-Reference

Vascular and Interventional Radiology: THE REQUISITES, p 402.

Comment

Although the cause of portal vein thrombosis remains undetermined in more than half of adult patients, commonly identifiable causes include hepatocellular carcinoma, cirrhosis, periportal inflammatory processes (e.g., pancreatitis, ascending cholangitis), and sepsis (the most common cause in children). Less-common causes include hypercoagulable states and trauma. Many patients are asymptomatic from the portal vein occlusion and present with symptoms of the underlying disease that caused the thrombosis. Despite the venous occlusion, hepatic failure and/or hepatomegaly are often not present.

Cross-sectional imaging modalities such as duplex ultrasound, helical CT, and MRI are fairly accurate in depicting portal vein thrombosis. In questionable cases, definitive diagnosis of acute or partial portal vein occlusion may be identified by observing a focal filling defect within the portal vein during the venous phase of a celiac or superior mesenteric arteriogram. With subacute or chronic portal venous thrombosis, large enhancing serpiginous collateral veins in the porta hepatis with nonvisualization of the normal expected portal venous branching pattern may be observed as in the image here, a finding known as *cavernous transformation of the portal vein.* Also important to observe in this image is the massively dilated vein that supplies a large gastroesophageal varix.

Notes

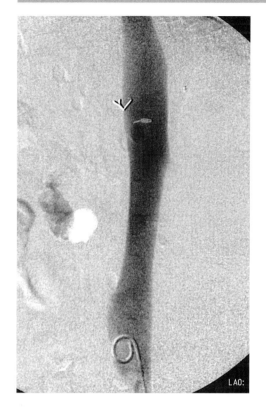

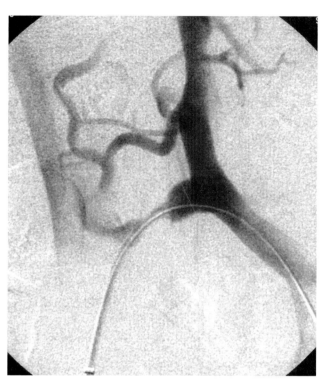

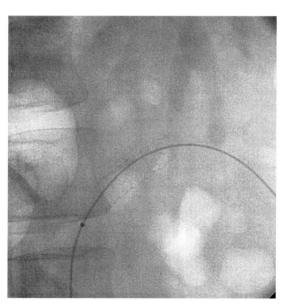

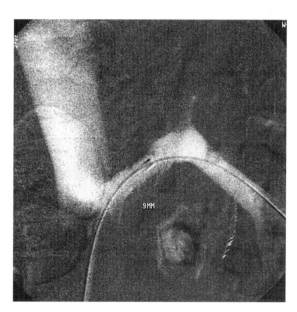

1. What surgical bypass procedure has been performed in this patient with hepatic cirrhosis, severe portal hypertension, and a history of variceal bleeding?

2. Why was the diagnostic study depicted in the first two images performed?

3. How was this study performed?

4. Does this study explain the presence of the clinical problems listed in Question 2?

Stenting of Mesocaval Shunt Stenosis

1. Mesocaval shunt.

2. Recurrent variceal bleeding or refractory ascites.

3. Placement of a catheter in the inferior vena cava (IVC) from a common femoral vein approach, catheterization of the shunt, superior mesenteric venography.

4. Yes. There is a tight stenosis in the mesocaval shunt (second image).

Reference

Zizka J, Elias P, Krajina A, et al. Value of Doppler sonography in revealing transjugular intrahepatic portosystemic shunt malfunction: A 5-year experience in 216 patients. *Am J Roentgenol*. 2000;175:141-148.

Cross-Reference

Vascular and Interventional Radiology: THE REQUISITES, pp 391-399.

Comment

Although transjugular intrahepatic portosystemic shunt (TIPS) placement is currently the most commonly used method of providing portal vein decompression in patients with symptomatic portal hypertension, a variety of surgical methods are occasionally used in these patients. Such options include the creation of a portacaval shunt (from main portal vein to IVC), a mesocaval shunt as shown here (from superior mesenteric vein to IVC), or a splenorenal shunt (from splenic vein to left renal vein). However, these conduits are also prone to develop stenosis and occlusion.

The images demonstrate catheterization of the mesocaval shunt from the IVC, with subsequent superior mesenteric venography. In this patient, recurrent variceal bleeding had occurred, and duplex ultrasound was unable to visualize the shunt. A tight stenosis was identified within the shunt. Angioplasty was performed initially but it did not produce a successful result, so a balloon-expandable Palmaz stent was placed within the shunt and dilated to 9 mm. An excellent venographic result is noted on the final image; this patient showed significant reduction of the mesocaval pressure gradient and experienced clinical success.

Notes

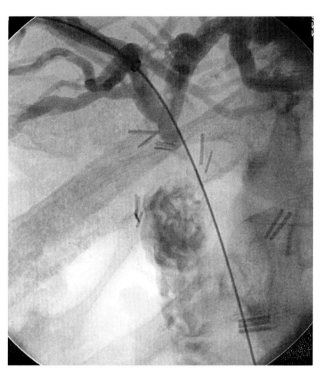

Courtesy of Dr. Daniel Brown.

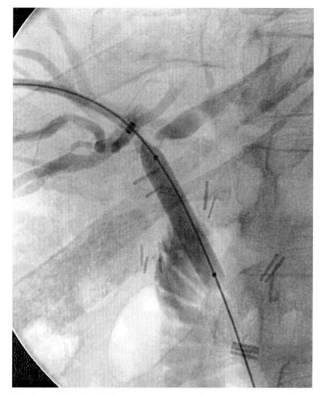

Courtesy of Dr. Daniel Brown.

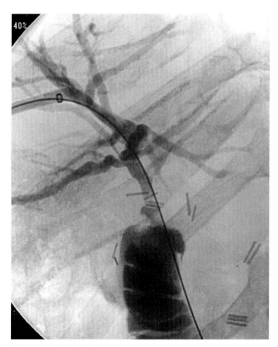

Courtesy of Dr. Daniel Brown.

1. What surgical procedure has been performed in this patient?

2. What symptoms might currently be present?

3. What abnormality is seen in the first image?

4. Is this typically treated with metallic biliary stent placement?

Biliary–Enteric Anastomotic Stricture

1. Hepaticojejunostomy.

2. Jaundice, cholangitis, elevated liver function tests.

3. Stenosis of the hepaticojejunostomy anastomosis.

4. No. Metallic stents are reserved for patients with malignant biliary obstruction and short life expectancy.

Reference

Laasch HU, Martin DF. Management of benign biliary strictures. *Cardiovasc Intervent Radiol.* 2002;25:457-466.

Cross-Reference

Vascular and Interventional Radiology: THE REQUISITES, pp 580-584.

Comment

A primary late complication of biliary surgery may be development of a stricture at the biliary–enteric anastomosis. Although surgical therapy can provide a durable treatment for this problem, the difficulty of performing repeat biliary surgery in the same operative bed is considerable. For this reason, percutaneous biliary drainage is usually performed initially. Balloon dilation of the anastomotic stricture can then be performed (final two images), and an internal–external drainage catheter can be left behind for several months to serve as a scaffold of good caliber around which the anastomosis can heal. Depending upon the results of balloon dilation, definitive surgical anastomotic revision might or might not be required.

Like other biliary interventions, antibiotic prophylaxis is recommended for biliary balloon dilation procedures. If the patient presents with cholangitis, then the balloon dilation procedure should be deferred to a future date when the patient is no longer infected. In this situation, at the initial sitting placement of a biliary drainage catheter should suffice.

Notes

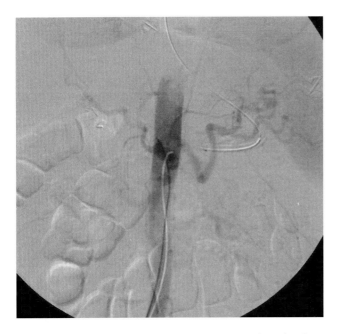 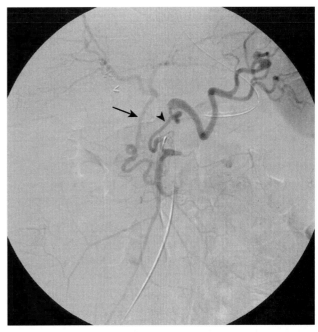

1. Which vessel is being selectively injected in the first image?

2. Which vessel is being selectively injected in the second image?

3. Name the arteries labeled by the arrow and arrowhead in the second image.

4. Which arteries are being filled by the two arteries named in question 3?

Anatomic Variant: Arc of Buhler

1. Celiac axis.

2. Superior mesenteric artery (SMA).

3. Gastroduodenal artery and the arc of Buhler, respectively.

4. The proper hepatic artery and the celiac axis, respectively.

Reference
Saad WE, Davies MG, Sahler L, et al. Arc of Buhler: Incidence and diameter in asymptomatic individuals. *Vasc Endovascular Surg*. 2005;39:347-349.

Cross-Reference
Vascular and Interventional Radiology: THE REQUISITES, p 291.

Comment
The celiac axis and the SMA develop from the 10th and 13th ventral segmental arteries off the aorta. The segmental arteries are connected by a ventral anastomosis that usually regresses during fetal development. Failure of regression results in a persistent arterial connection called the arc of Buhler. This acts as a collateral pathway between the celiac axis and the SMA, which can become a critical finding to identify in patients with celiac axis or SMA stenosis and in patients undergoing transarterial chemoembolization, hepatic artery radioembolization, pancreaticoduodenal surgeries, or liver transplantation.

Notes

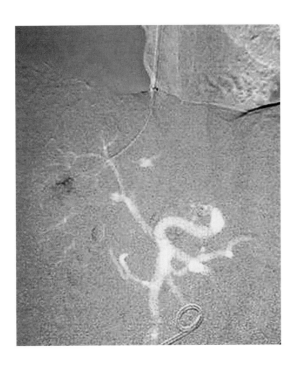
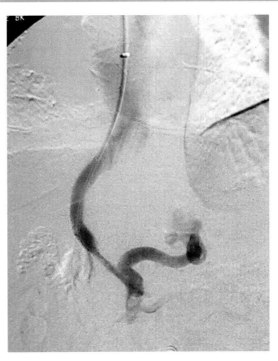

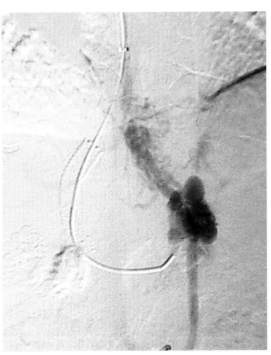

1. How was the first image obtained?

2. After placement of a transjugular intrahepatic portosystemic shunt (TIPS), what residual abnormality is seen in the third image?

3. What procedure was performed to treat this abnormality?

4. Can this procedure be expected to be effective in preventing variceal bleeding in the absence of preceding TIPS placement?

Post-TIPS Variceal Embolization

1. Wedged carbon dioxide portography via a hepatic vein balloon catheter.

2. Large bleeding gastroesophageal varix.

3. Coil embolization of the varix.

4. No.

Reference

Hidajat N, Stobbe H, Hosten N, et al. Transjugular intrahepatic portosystemic shunt and transjugular embolization of bleeding rectal varices in portal hypertension. *Am J Roentgenol.* 2002;178:362-363.

Cross-Reference

Vascular and Interventional Radiology: THE REQUISITES, pp 391-399.

Comment

The hemodynamic goal of TIPS is to achieve the optimal degree of reduction in the portosystemic gradient thatwill prevent variceal bleeding and ascites but that will preserve hepatic perfusion (thereby preventing encephalopathy and liver failure). In most patients, reducing the portosystemic gradient to 8 to 12 mm Hg produces this effect. Likewise, in most patients, portal venography performed immediately after TIPS demonstrates markedly reduced filling of gastroesophageal varices compared to the pre-TIPS venogram. In a minority of patients, however, persistent variceal filling is observed (second and third images).

When this occurs, the presence of residual stenosis or thrombus within the TIPS tract or portal vein should first be sought and corrected by additional angioplasty or stent placement. If variceal filling is still observed, or in select cases in which the patient is hemodynamically unstable due to variceal bleeding, the gastroesophageal varices can be selected from the portal venous system and percutaneously embolized using coils.

Notes

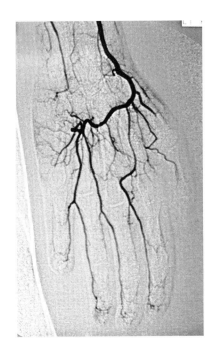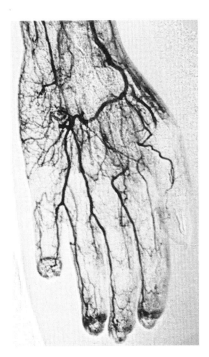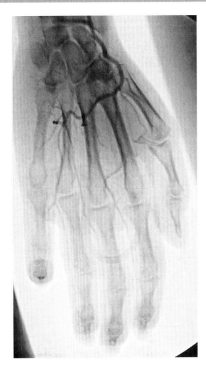

1. What vascular abnormalities are seen?

2. Name four potential causes of these findings.

3. What is the underlying diagnosis in this patient?

4. How can one determine if a significant vasospastic component is present?

Scleroderma

1. Multiple occlusions and stenoses in the palmar and digital arteries.

2. Emboli, vasculitis, traumatic lesions, vasospasm.

3. Scleroderma.

4. Angiography following infusion of a vasodilator.

Reference

Stucker M, Quinna S, Memmel U, et al. Macroangiopathy of the upper extremities in progressive systemic sclerosis. *Eur J Med Res*. 2000;5(7):295-302.

Cross-Reference

Vascular and Interventional Radiology: THE REQUISITES, p 147.

Comment

Small artery occlusions and stenoses in the palmar and digital arteries can produce severe pain, paresthesias, Raynaud's phenomenon, fingertip necrosis, and gangrene. The pathophysiology of vascular lesions in these patients often includes embolic, traumatic, vasoreactive, and inflammatory components. Diagnostic evaluation should focus upon identifying contributing factors that are treatable by medical or surgical interventions.

First, the angiogram should be carefully scrutinized for any evidence of emboli. Potential sources of digital emboli include the heart (diagnosed by echocardiography and treated with anticoagulation), atherosclerotic plaques in the subclavian artery (treated with anticoagulation and/or surgical removal of the source lesion), sports-related injury to the axillary artery (subject to surgical repair), and occupational vascular injuries such as hypothenar hammer syndrome (also subject to surgical repair). Second, the presence of a significant vasospastic component to the arterial lesions should be sought during the angiographic evaluation. If the stenotic lesions improve significantly following administration of a vasodilator (such as tolazoline or nitroglycerine), then a sympathectomy may be more likely to provide some degree of symptom relief.

Unfortunately, this patient has irreversible small-vessel occlusions due to scleroderma. The vascular findings mimic those seen with other small-vessel diseases. However, the diagnosis of scleroderma can confidently be made in this patient due to the clear radiographic evidence of acro-osteolysis (final image).

Notes

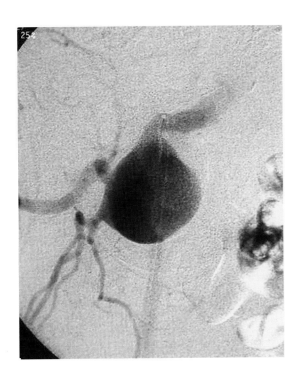

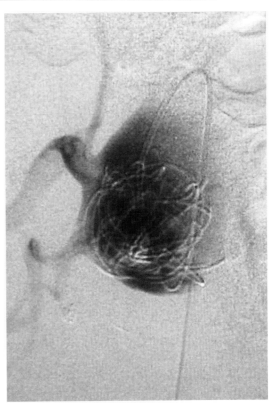

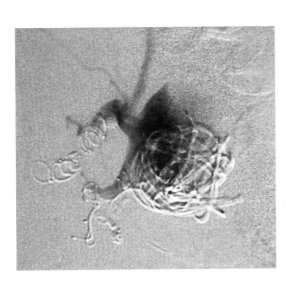

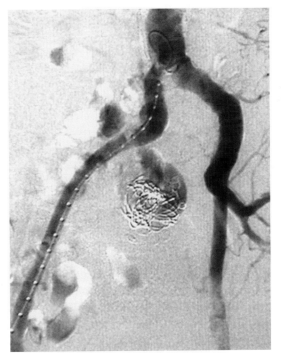

1. What is the diagnosis?

2. For asymptomatic lesions, what diameter mandates surgical treatment?

3. What factors make surgical treatment of this lesion complex?

4. Will embolization alone provide effective therapy?

Internal Iliac Artery Aneurysm

1. Right internal iliac artery aneurysm.

2. From 3.0 to 3.5 cm in diameter and larger.

3. Location deep within the pelvis, proximity to the ureter, multiple outflow vessels.

4. No. Embolization has been performed to occlude the outflow vessels of the lesion. A stent graft will be placed in the right iliac artery to occlude its inflow.

References

Sanchez LA, Patel AV, Ohki T, et al. Midterm experience with the endovascular treatment of isolated iliac aneurysms. *J Vasc Surg.* 1999;30:907-914.

Razavi MK, Dake MD, Semba CP, et al. Percutaneous endoluminal placement of stent-grafts for the treatment of isolated iliac artery aneurysms. *Radiology.* 1995;197:801-804.

Cross-Reference

Vascular and Interventional Radiology: THE REQUISITES, pp 252-261.

Comment

Isolated iliac artery aneurysms can rupture, embolize, or produce local compression symptoms. The rate of rupture increases significantly between 3 and 4 cm, and therefore most surgeons recommend operative repair for iliac aneurysms larger than 3.0 to 3.5 cm in diameter. Because retroperitoneal dissection can be difficult when the aneurysm morphology is complex, endovascular methods to repair iliac aneurysms have gained favor in recent years. So far, the primary patencies of stent grafts for iliac artery aneurysms have been excellent (92%-100% at 1-4 years), and the incidence of endoleaks has been very low.

Because of the late potential for cross-pelvic collaterals to reconstitute the aneurysm sac, it is very important to gain control of all distal vessels arising from the aneurysm, either by surgical ligation or by coil embolization (shown in the last three images). Once these outflow vessels are successfully occluded, the inflow to the aneurysm may be occluded by placing a stent graft across the origin of the internal iliac artery. The final image shows a marker catheter in the right iliac artery being used to measure the iliac artery to appropriately size the stent-graft device to be used.

Notes

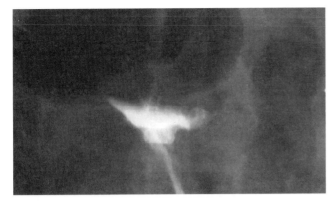

Courtesy of Dr. David Hovsepian.

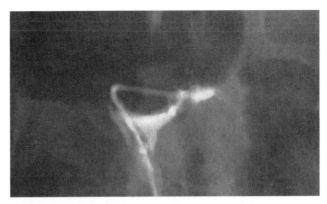

Courtesy of Dr. David Hovsepian.

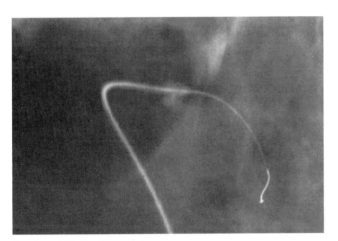

Courtesy of Dr. David Hovsepian.

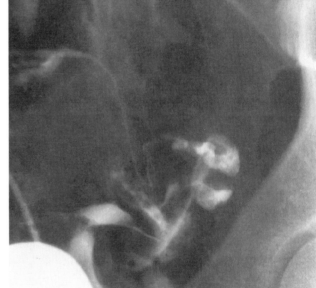

Courtesy of Dr. David Hovsepian.

1. What examination is depicted in the first image?

2. What examination is depicted in the second image?

3. Why are these examinations being performed?

4. What diagnosis is evident on the first two images?

Fallopian Tube Recanalization

1. Nonselective hysterosalpingogram (HSG).

2. Selective salpingography.

3. To evaluate and treat female infertility caused by proximal tubal occlusion.

4. Bilateral proximal fallopian tube occlusions.

Reference

Pinto AB, Hovsepian DM, Wattanakumtornkul S, et al. Pregnancy outcomes after fallopian tube recanalization: oil-based versus water-soluble contrast agents. *J Vasc Interv Radiol.* 2003;14:69-74.

Cross-Reference

Vascular and Interventional Radiology: THE REQUI-SITES, pp 602-635.

Comment

HSG is commonly performed in the evaluation of female-factor infertility. Several causes of infertility may be detected by HSG, including congenital uterine anomalies (which are also well depicted by MRI), extrinsic uterine cavity distortion by mass lesions (commonly fibroids or adenomyosis), Asherman's syndrome (filling defects representing intrauterine septations may be visualized on HSG), salpingitis isthmica nodosa (pelvic inflammatory disease–related scarring and tubal occlusion), and proximal tubal occlusion.

When the nonselective HSG depicts proximal tubal occlusion (first image), a small catheter may be used to select the orifice of the fallopian tube (second image). If tubal occlusion is confirmed, as in this case, a guidewire may be gently advanced beyond the occlusion in an attempt to dislodge an occlusive mucus plug (third image). Repeat salpingogram then demonstrates spill of contrast into the peritoneal cavity, consistent with a patent (recanalized) fallopian tube (final image).

Fallopian tube recanalization restores patency to at least one tube in approximately 80% of patients, and it has been shown to significantly improve pregnancy rates.

Notes

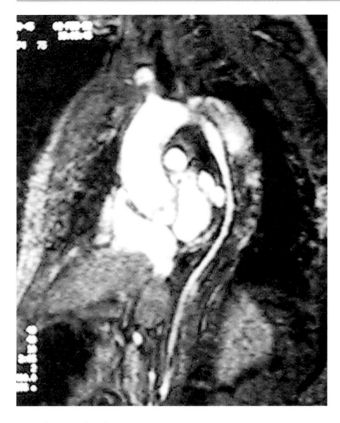

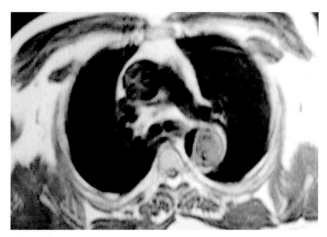

1. What is the diagnosis?

2. What complication appears to be present?

3. Is MRI more sensitive and specific than aortography for this diagnosis?

4. What other modalities are equally sensitive and specific for this diagnosis?

MRI of Aortic Dissection

1. Aortic dissection.

2. True lumen collapse.

3. Yes.

4. Helical CT and multiplanar transesophageal echocardiography (TEE).

Reference

Moore AG, Eagle KA, Bruckman D, et al. Choice of computed tomography, transesophageal echocardiography, magnetic resonance imaging, and aortography in acute aortic dissection: International Registry of Acute Aortic Dissection (IRAD). *Am J Cardiol.* 2002;89: 1235-1238.

Cross-Reference

Vascular and Interventional Radiology: THE REQUISITES, pp 223-228.

Comment

The images in this case clearly visualize an aortic dissection flap extending throughout the descending thoracic aorta. The diameter of the true lumen is noted to be extremely small throughout the descending thoracic aorta.

MRI is equal or superior to helical CT and TEE for making the diagnosis of acute and chronic aortic dissection. The longer image-acquisition time and greater difficulty in patient monitoring in the MRI scanner have been considered relative disadvantages of its use in the acute aortic dissection setting. However, MRI and helical CT are better able than TEE to evaluate the entire aorta (including its subdiaphragmatic segment), and MRI has the advantage in not requiring iodinated contrast.

All three cross-sectional modalities are significantly superior to aortography for making the diagnosis of aortic dissection. In current practice, aortography is reserved for evaluating patients with clinical evidence of complications of aortic dissection for whom surgical or interventional therapy is being planned.

Notes

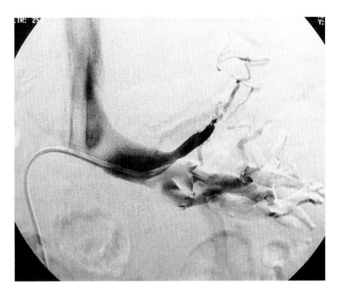
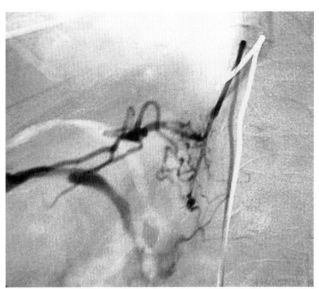

1. What procedure is being performed?

2. What endocrine condition might this patient have?

3. What specific information can this procedure provide?

4. What is Conn's syndrome?

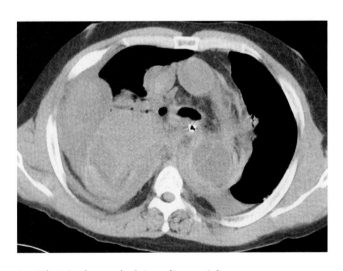
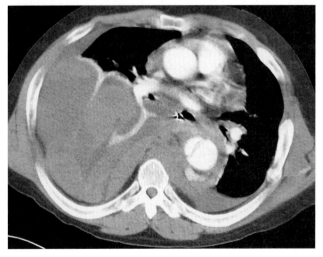

1. What is the underlying diagnosis?

2. What complication is seen?

3. What is the appropriate clinical management of this problem?

4. If peripheral ischemic symptoms are present, is this patient a candidate for percutaneous fenestration of the aortic flap?

Selective Adrenal Vein Sampling

1. Bilateral selective adrenal venography.

2. Primary hyperaldosteronism.

3. Measurement of aldosterone level can help to localize an adrenal adenoma.

4. Hypertension due to an aldosterone-producing adrenal adenoma.

Reference

Wheeler MH, Harris DA. Diagnosis and management of primary aldosteronism. *World J Surg.* 2003;27: 627-631.

Cross-Reference

Vascular and Interventional Radiology: THE REQUISITES, pp 374-375.

Comment

Primary aldosteronism is important to identify within the hypertensive population, because most patients with a unilateral source of excess aldosterone production are amenable to surgical cure. Typically, postural hormonal testing is first performed by an endocrinologist. The diagnosis is then confirmed by selective adrenal venous sampling with measurement of aldosterone concentrations (expressed as aldosterone-to-cortisol ratio) in each adrenal vein. Selective adrenal venous sampling has been shown to be more sensitive and specific than cross-sectional imaging or scintigraphy, and endocrine surgeons are often guided by the results of the sampling study. Patients with unilateral disease are ideally treated by laparoscopic adrenalectomy. Patients in whom localization is not achieved usually have bilateral adrenal hyperplasia and are treated medically.

Aortic Dissection with Rupture

1. Aortic dissection.

2. Rupture of the thoracic aorta with bilateral hemothorax.

3. Emergency surgical thoracic aortic replacement.

4. No. This patient needs emergency aortic surgery.

Reference

Marty-Ane CH, Berthet JP, Branchereau P, et al. Endovascular repair for acute traumatic rupture of the thoracic aorta. *Ann Thorac Surg.* 2003;75:1803-1807.

Cross-Reference

Vascular and Interventional Radiology: THE REQUISITES, pp 235-239.

Comment

Aortic rupture is a dreaded complication of aortic dissection. Stanford type A dissections carry a moderate risk of ascending aortic rupture into the pericardial sac, producing pericardial tamponade; to prevent this, these patients are treated with immediate aortic repair. Stanford type B dissections typically are managed medically, and they only occasionally progress to aortic rupture. Clinical signs that can indicate impending or completed aortic rupture are persistent or increasing chest pain, uncontrolled hypertension, the development of a left pleural effusion on chest radiography or CT, and/or hemodynamic instability. In the case shown here, aortic rupture with bilateral hemothorax is clearly depicted on both noncontrast and contrast-enhanced CT.

The standard of care for the treatment of aortic rupture is immediate surgical aortic replacement. Recently, in a small number of centers, stable patients with ruptured aortic dissections and aneurysms have been managed using endovascular stent-graft repair. The main potential advantage of this innovative approach is the ability to avoid thoracotomy and aortic clamping in this subset of patients who tend to have multiple comorbidities. However, aortic stent-graft placement for such high-risk patients has not yet been validated in comparative trials. Early results for aortic stent-graft placement have been encouraging, and it is being used as an alternative to open surgical repair at an increasing rate.

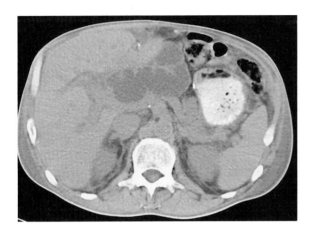
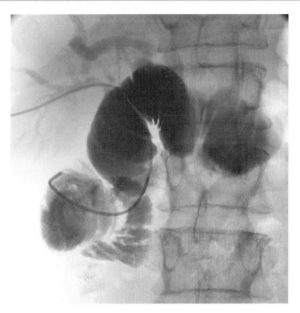

1. What is the etiology of biliary dilation in this patient who has previously undergone a Whipple procedure with hepaticojejunosomy and Roux-en-Y?

2. What symptoms might this patient present with?

3. What procedure can be initially performed to palliate these symptoms?

4. Name two anatomic approaches to this procedure.

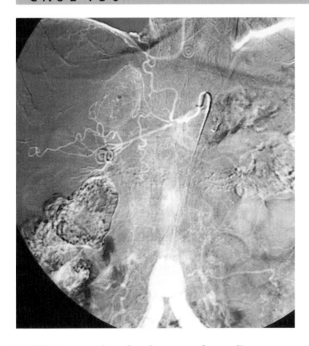
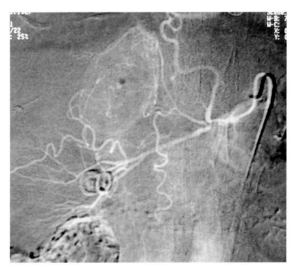

1. What procedure has been performed?

2. What abnormality is seen?

3. Is this likely to be malignant?

4. How would this likely be treated?

CASE 149

Afferent Loop Obstruction

1. Afferent loop syndrome.

2. Abdominal pain, increasing jaundice, possibly cholangitis.

3. Placement of a decompressive drainage catheter within the afferent loop.

4. Transhepatic biliary route, direct transabdominal route into the loop itself.

Reference

Gayer G, Barsuk D, Hertz M, et al. CT diagnosis of afferent loop syndrome. *Clin Radiol*. 2002;57:835-839.

Cross-Reference

Vascular and Interventional Radiology: THE REQUISITES, pp 537-539.

Comment

The first image demonstrates bilateral biliary dilation and severe dilation of a loop of bowel that courses into the hepatic hilum. In the setting of abdominal symptoms and a known Whipple procedure, the possibility of an afferent loop obstruction must be considered. Decompression of this loop can be accomplished surgically (usually reserved for patients in whom the hepaticojejunostomy was performed for benign disease) or via percutaneous placement of a drainage catheter within the dilated loop (second image). Once initial decompression has occurred, if a stenosis at the bowel–bowel anastomosis is detected and the patient has short life expectancy, then a metallic stent may be placed within the stenosis to relieve the obstruction in carefully selected patients.

CASE 150

Adrenal Adenoma

1. Selective right adrenal arteriogram.

2. Right adrenal mass lesion.

3. No, but one cannot be sure based upon angiography alone.

4. Surgical adrenalectomy with or without preoperative embolization.

Reference

Blake MA, Jhaveri KS, Sweeney AT, et al. State of the art in adrenal imaging. *Curr Probl Diagn Radiol*. 2002;31(3):67-78.

Cross-Reference

Vascular and Interventional Radiology: THE REQUISITES, pp 346-347.

Comment

These images demonstrate a selective right adrenal arteriogram. Although the arterial supply to the adrenal gland can vary, one common arrangement has three main arteries supplying the gland: an inferior adrenal artery derived from the ipsilateral renal artery, a middle adrenal artery derived from the aorta, and a superior adrenal artery derived from the inferior phrenic artery.

In the case presented, a well-defined, enhancing mass is identified in the right adrenal gland. The angiographic appearance favors a benign etiology such as an adenoma (which is what this was). Angiographic features that might suggest malignancy can include more prominent hypervascularity, arteriovenous shunting, neovascularity, recruitment of arterial supply from multiple vessels, and lack of clearly defined borders.

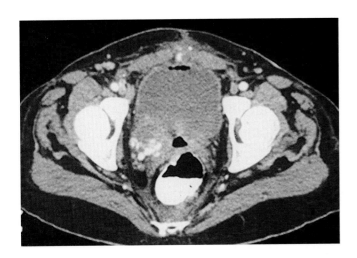
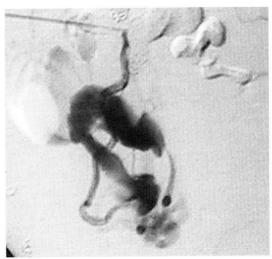
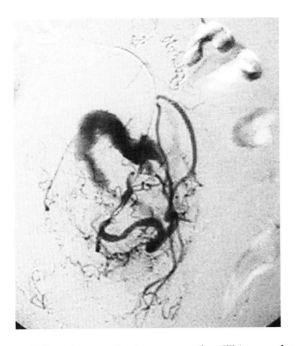
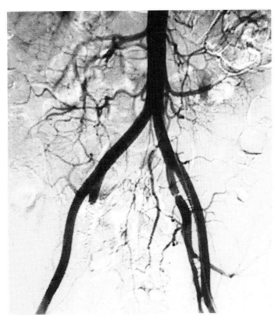

1. What abnormality is seen on the CT image above?

2. What artery is catheterized in the second and third images?

3. What is the diagnosis?

4. How might this be treated?

Uterine Arteriovenous Malformation

1. Multiple enhancing vascular structures in the right hemipelvis.

2. Right uterine artery.

3. Arteriovenous malformation (AVM) of the pelvis.

4. Sequential arterial embolization procedures.

Reference

Gulati MS, Paul SB, Batra A, et al. Uterine arteriovenous malformations: The role of intravenous "dual-phase" CT angiography. *Clin Imaging.* 2000;24(1):10-14.

Cross-Reference

Vascular and Interventional Radiology: THE REQUISITES, pp 280-282.

Comment

Life-threatening vaginal bleeding can be caused by a variety of hypervascular masses, including uterine fibroids, gestational trophoblastic disease, cervical carcinoma and other pelvic malignancies, ectopic pregnancies, and AVM. In the case presented here, injection of the uterine artery reveals a tortuous collection of arteries with early opacification of a large draining vein, consistent with a uterine AVM. Embolization was performed, and the final image shows internal iliac artery occlusion.

Uterine AVMs are rare lesions; they can be congenital or acquired. Previous uterine surgery or curettage, uterine trauma, past history of gestational trophoblastic disease, previous pregnancy, genital tract malignancy, and diethylstilbestrol exposure are all predisposing factors associated with acquired uterine AVMs. Although hysterectomy has long been considered the treatment of choice for these lesions, embolization therapy is now used for women wishing to retain their fertility.

Unlike AVMs that are confined to the uterus, curative treatment of extrauterine pelvic AVMs is rarely possible because pelvic organ involvement and complex arterial supply render surgical resection hazardous. Sequential embolization therapy can be used for these patients to palliate symptoms and limit the frequency and severity of recurrent bleeding. Unfortunately, recurrence rates are high despite embolization.

Notes

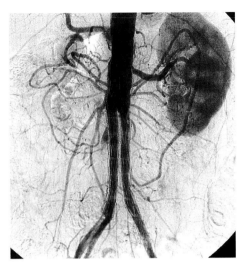

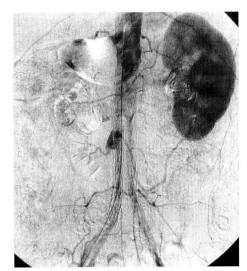

Courtesy of Dr. David Hovsepian.　　Courtesy of Dr. David Hovsepian.

1. Is angiography the primary method of follow-up for patients who have undergone endoluminal aortic aneurysm repair?

2. What abnormality is seen in the images above?

3. If this aneurysm is increasing in size, does this abnormality require treatment?

4. Would this be treated by insertion of an additional stent graft?

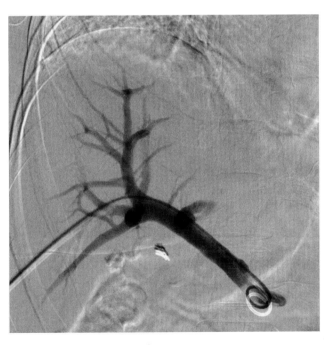

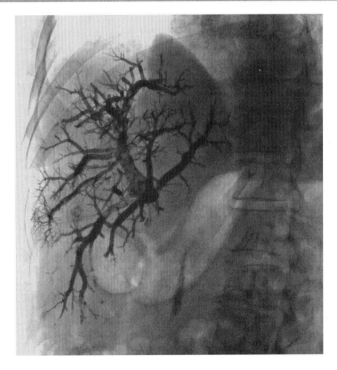

1. What examination is being performed in the first image?

2. What intervention has been performed in the second image?

3. What embolic agent has been used?

4. What are the indications for performing this procedure?

C A S E 1 5 2

Type II Endoleak

1. No. CT scanning is the primary follow-up method.

2. Type II endoleak via retrograde flow in a lumbar artery.

3. Yes.

4. No.

Reference

Faries PL, Cadot H, Agarwal G, et al. Management of endoleak after endovascular aneurysm repair: Cuffs, coils, and conversion. *J Vasc Surg.* 2003;37(1): 1155-1161.

Cross-Reference

Vascular and Interventional Radiology: THE REQUI-SITES, pp 256-260.

Comment

Patients who undergo endoluminal repair of abdominal aortic aneurysms (AAA) typically receive close surveillance with periodic CT angiography. When extraluminal contrast is seen within the aneurysm sac on CT, the presence of an endoleak is confirmed. Precise characterization of the type and etiology of endoleak is critical in planning treatment and usually requires angiography. These images demonstrate a collection of contrast in the right aspect of the aneurysm sac, which is clearly being fed by retrograde flow in a lumbar artery (second image). Contrast does not enter the aneurysm sac in the early arterial phase (first image), as would typically be seen with a type I (attachment site) endoleak.

Patients with type II endoleaks and evidence of aneurysm enlargment on serial CT scans require treatment due to the risk of aneurysm rupture. The criteria upon which to base treatment of type II endoleaks in the absence of aneurysm enlargement are highly controversial, in part because more than 50% tend to close spontaneously. Hence, some physicians treat all type II leaks, some treat only endoleaks that are first detected several months after the procedure, and others believe that close CT follow-up is sufficient.

C A S E 1 5 3

Portal Vein Embolization

1. Percutaneous transhepatic portal venography.

2. Selective right portal vein embolization.

3. *N*-Butyl cyanoacrylate (NBCA) mixed with ethiodol.

4. To induce hypertrophy of the future liver remnant (FLR) before hepatic resection.

Reference

Madoff DC, Hicks ME, Vauthey JN, et al. Transhepatic portal vein embolization: Anatomy, indications, and technical considerations. *Radiographics.* 2002;22: 1063-1076.

Cross-Reference

Vascular and Interventional Radiology: THE REQUI-SITES, pp 215-217.

Comment

Major hepatic resection is being performed at an increasing rate in the treatment of primary and secondary hepatobiliary malignancy. One of the potential postoperative complications associated with this type of surgery is fatal liver failure. This can result from the inability of the remaining liver parenchyma after resection to provide adequate function to sustain life. Preresection measures to increase the volume of the FLR have been employed to make some patients eligible for this type of surgery. This has been achieved by surgical ligation of the contralateral portal vein in the past, and more recently it is achieved with contralateral portal vein embolization (PVE).

Preprocedural cross-sectional imaging is obtained to evaluate the total liver volume (TLV) and the estimated FLR volume. A FLV/TLV ratio of 20% to 40% is recommended for patients before planned major hepatic resection. An ipsilateral or contralateral approach is used. Various embolic materials have been used for PVE including NBCA, polyvinyl alcohol (PVA) particles, Gelfoam, and coils. Follow-up cross-sectional imaging with calculation of the liver volume is obtained in 2 to 4 weeks to assess the degree of FLR hypertrophy.

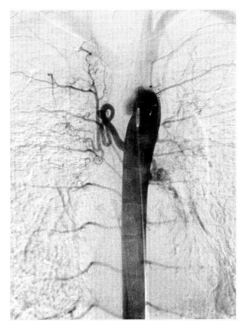

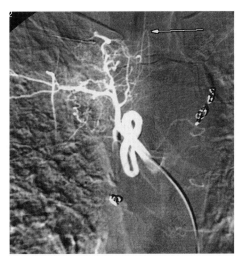

Courtesy of Dr. James Duncan.   Courtesy of Dr. James Duncan.

1. What examination has been performed in the second image?

2. What artery is marked by the arrow in the second image?

3. From what vessel does this artery arise?

4. Is visualization of this vessel a contraindication to bronchial embolization?

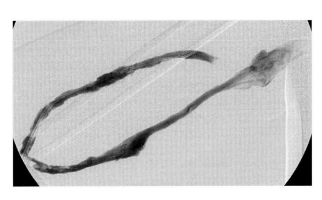

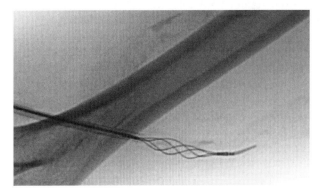

1. What study is depicted in the first image?

2. Based upon the appearance of the graft apex region in the first image (which is mid-procedure), what problem may have prompted this examination?

3. What treatment options are available for occluded dialysis grafts?

4. What treatment method is depicted in the second image?

C A S E 1 5 4

Spinal Artery

1. Selective right bronchial arteriogram.

2. A spinal artery.

3. From the very proximal right bronchial artery.

4. No. However, the catheter needs to be positioned well distal to the origin of that branch before embolization to prevent reflux of embolic material into that branch.

Reference

Tanaka N, Yamakado K, Murashima S, et al. Superselective bronchial artery embolization for hemoptysis with a coaxial microcatheter system. *J Vasc Interv Radiol.* 1997;8(1 Pt 1):65-70.

Cross-Reference

Vascular and Interventional Radiology: THE REQUISITES, pp 215-217.

Comment

The first image, a descending thoracic aortogram, demonstrates an enlarged right bronchial artery in a patient being evaluated for hemoptysis. In the second image, a selective right bronchial arteriogram, a tortuous bronchial artery is seen. Importantly, a spinal artery is seen to arise from the proximal aspect of the right bronchial artery. The vessel takes a characteristic hairpin turn before entering the vertebral canal to supply the spinal cord.

Identification of spinal arteries during bronchial arteriography is important in avoiding the complication of paraplegia. Also, whereas in the past embolization was performed from the main bronchial artery through a 4- to 5-F catheter placed in the proximal segment of the bronchial artery, most interventionalists now place a microcatheter distally in the bronchial artery in order to avoid nontarget embolization of any proximal spinal or intercostal branches that may be present. For these reasons, the incidence of neurologic complications following bronchial arteriography is extremely low.

C A S E 1 5 5

Thrombosed Dialysis Graft

1. Dialysis fistulogram.

2. Graft thrombosis.

3. Percutaneous declotting of the graft, surgical thrombectomy.

4. A mechanical thrombectomy device (the percutaneous thrombolytic device).

Reference

Vesely TM. Mechanical thrombectomy devices to treat thrombosed hemodialysis grafts. *Tech Vasc Interv Radiol.* 2003;6(1):35-41.

Cross-Reference

Vascular and Interventional Radiology: THE REQUISITES, pp 184-191.

Comment

A dialysis graft is a surgically created arteriovenous fistula using prosthetic materials to the bridge the gap between an artery and a vein. There are a variety of configurations, with the most common being loop grafts in the forearm and C grafts in the upper arm.

Because the outflow veins are exposed to "arterial" pressures and flows, and because of the frequent needle punctures needed for dialysis, dialysis grafts are prone to eventual failure. This failure can manifest by high venous pressures during dialysis sessions, excessive bleeding from the puncture sites, arm swelling, high recirculation values, or, ultimately, graft thrombosis.

The goals of treatment are to clear the thrombus from the graft and to treat the underlying cause of the thrombosis. Thrombus may be cleared by percutaneous declotting using pharmacologic thrombolysis or a mechanical thrombectomy device (second image). The underlying cause of graft thrombosis is diagnosed by venography performed during the percutaneous declotting procedure, and it is typically treated using angioplasty and/or stent placement. Unfortunately, a thrombosed graft with completely occluded outflow veins or long-segment stricture of these veins might not be amenable to percutaneous re-establishment of flow. In these cases, surgical revision or creation of new access may be necessary.

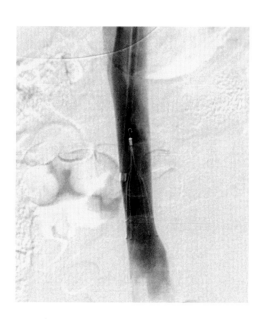 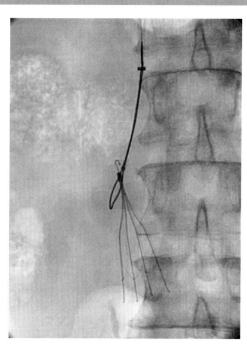

1. What type of inferior vena cava (IVC) filter is shown?

2. Why is there a hook at the upper end of the filter?

3. Besides the filter, what device is pictured in the second image?

4. Why is this filter being removed?

Retrievable Inferior Vena Cava Filter

1. Günther Tulip.

2. To enable percutaneous removal.

3. Amplatz Goose Neck Snare (Microvena).

4. The risk of pulmonary embolism is probably significantly diminished compared with when the filter was placed.

Reference

Kinney TB. Update on inferior vena cava filters. *J Vasc Intervent Radiol.* 2003;14:425-440.

Cross-Reference

Vascular and Interventional Radiology: THE REQUISITES, pp 364-368.

Comment

The images picture a Günther Tulip (Cook) filter, which is well positioned within the infrarenal IVC. This filter is percutaneously retrievable by snaring the upper hook, provided no thrombus is present within the filter. Particular subsets of patients in whom these filters might be useful include trauma patients and postoperative patients who have a reason to be hypercoagulable for a defined period of time (e.g. hip surgery or abdominal-perineal resection patients).

Currently approved filters in the United States include three types of Greenfield filter (stainless steel, titanium, and over-the-wire), VenaTech filter, bird's nest filter, Simon nitinol filter, Trap Ease filter, OptEase filter, G2 filter, and the Tulip pictured here. There are few convincing data to demonstrate the superiority of any particular filter.

Notes

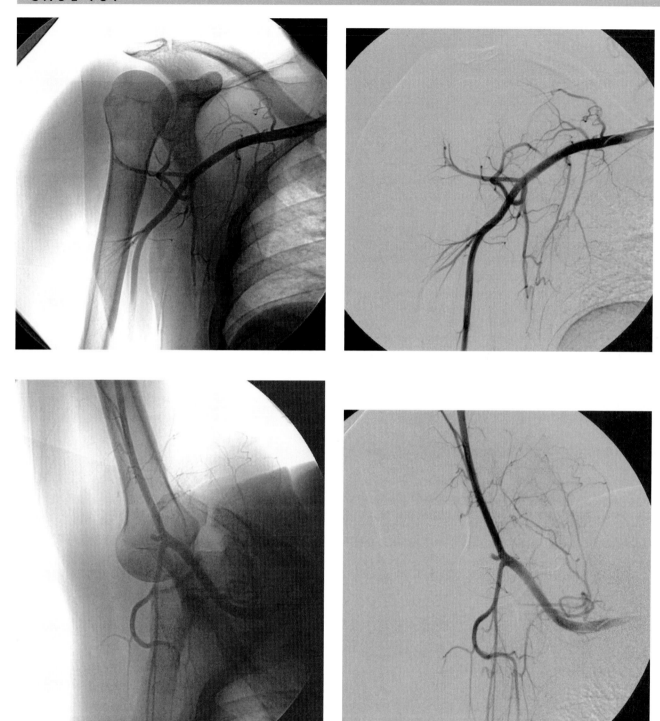

1. What procedure is being performed in the first two images?

2. What abnormal finding is seen in the second two images?

3. What provocative maneuver was performed to elicit this finding?

4. What is the diagnosis?

Quadrilateral Space Syndrome

1. Selective right upper extremity arteriography.

2. Abrupt occlusion of the posterior humeral circumflex artery.

3. Hyperabduction of the shoulder.

4. Quadrilateral space syndrome.

References

Mochizuki T, Isoda H, Masui T, et al. Occlusion of the posterior humeral circumflex artery: Detection with MR angiography in healthy volunteers and in a patient with quadrilateral space syndrome. *AJR Am J Roentgenol.* 1994;163:625-627.

Cormier PJ, Matalon TA, Wolin PM. Quadrilateral space syndrome: A rare cause of shoulder pain. *Radiology.* 1998;167:797-798.

Comment

The quadrilateral space is bounded by the teres minor superiorly, the surgical neck of the humerus laterally, the long head of the triceps medially, and the upper border of the teres major inferiorly. It contains the axillary nerve and the posterior circumflex humeral artery. Quadrilateral space syndrome is a rare condition in which the contents of the quadrilateral space are compressed, leading to vague symptoms of shoulder pain, tenderness over the quadrilateral space on palpation, and teres minor and deltoid denervation.

The most commonly cited cause of compression of quadrilateral space structures is fibrous bands. Other causes include glenoid labral cysts, a ganglion, muscle hypertrophy, and a spike of bone after a scapular fracture.

The prevalence of quadrilateral space syndrome is unknown. On angiography, a position of abduction and external rotation demonstrates significant compression of the contents of the quadrilateral space. Nerve conduction studies and electromyography have also been used to investigate quadrilateral space syndrome. The appearance of denervation changes on MRI affecting the teres minor muscle is considered to confirm the diagnosis of quadrilateral space syndrome. Treatment is centered on surgical decompression of the contents of the quadrilateral space.

Notes

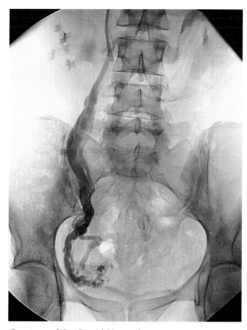

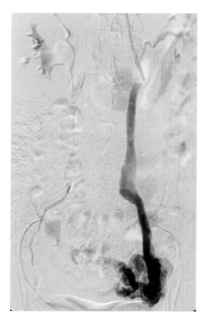

Courtesy of Dr. David Hovsepian.   Courtesy of Dr. David Hovsepian.

1. In order, what veins were catheterized to obtain the first image?

2. In order, what veins were catheterized to obtain the second image?

3. What symptom is this woman likely to present with?

4. What procedure can be performed to treat the symptom?

Pelvic Congestion Syndrome

1. Inferior vena cava, right ovarian vein.

2. Inferior vena cava, left renal vein, left ovarian vein.

3. Chronic pelvic pain.

4. Ovarian and internal iliac vein embolization.

Reference

Venbrux AC, Chang AH, Kim HS, et al. Pelvic congestion syndrome (pelvic venous incompetence): Impact of ovarian and internal iliac vein embolotherapy on menstrual cycle and chronic pelvic pain. *J Vasc Intervent Radiol*. 2002;13(2 Pt 1):171-178.

Cross-Reference

Vascular and Interventional Radiology: THE REQUISITES, pp 372-373.

Comment

Chronic pelvic pain can result from problems in the reproductive organs or it may be neurologic, musculoskeletal, urologic, or gastrointestinal in nature. However, the association of ovarian and pelvic varices with chronic pelvic pain has been known for many years. Pelvic venous incompetence may be suspected when a woman reports pelvic pain in the upright position, during or after intercourse, or when varicosities are visualized in the thigh, buttocks, or perineum.

Analogous to a male varicocele, ovarian and pelvic varices are amenable to treatment by transcatheter embolization of the refluxing ovarian veins. For this procedure, each ovarian vein is catheterized and examined with venography to determine whether significant reflux is present. If it is, the ovarian vein and internal iliac vein are embolized. Embolization of the internal iliac vein is recommended because of the well-documented communications between the ovarian veins and the internal iliac veins. Embolization therapy may be expected to produce some degree of symptomatic improvement in 70% to 90% of women undergoing the procedure, provided a rigorous clinical and imaging screening process is used to select patients initially.

Notes

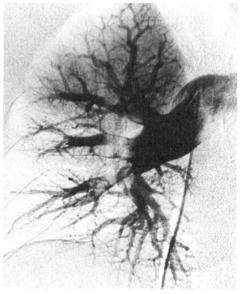

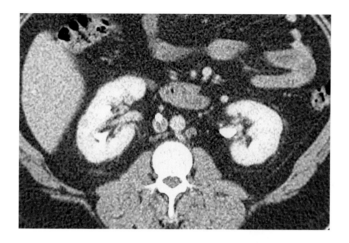

Courtesy of Dr. James Duncan.

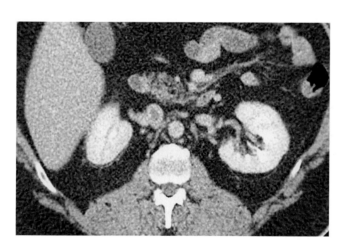

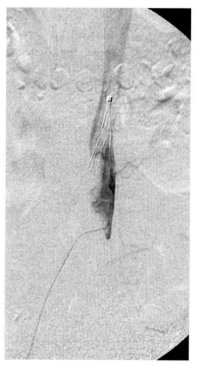

1. What is the diagnosis in the first image?

2. Is this finding acute or chronic?

3. What possible explanations exist for pulmonary embolism in the presence of an inferior vena cava (IVC) filter?

4. What is the explanation in this patient?

Inferior Vena Cava Filter Failure

1. Pulmonary embolism.

2. Acute.

3. IVC filter thrombosis may be present, a collateral pathway around the filter may be present, upper extremity venous thrombosis may have embolized.

4. IVC filter thrombosis (second image) with thrombus extension above the filter (third and fourth images).

Reference

Streiff MB. Vena caval filters: A comprehensive review. *Blood*. 2000;95:3669-3677.

Cross-Reference

Vascular and Interventional Radiology: THE REQUISITES, pp 364-368.

Comment

Inferior vena cava filters are associated with a 2% to 4% annual rate of recurrent pulmonary embolism. There are several reasons this is the case. First, being a metallic intravascular foreign body, the filter itself can predispose to IVC thrombosis in hypercoagulable patients. If this occurs and any thrombus extends above the filter (as in this case), pulmonary embolism can occur. Second, the filter material simply might not prevent small emboli from slipping through. Third, if the filter was not positioned below the lowest renal vein, accessory pathways can provide a route for emboli from the lower-extremity veins to bypass the filter. Fourth, large venous collaterals or a duplicated inferior vena cava (if not identified on initial venography) can rarely provide a similar bypass route for emboli. Fifth, malpositioned filters, excessively angulated filters, and the rare filter that migrates might not be in proper position to catch emboli.

For these reasons, when pulmonary embolism occurs despite IVC filter placement, repeat inferior vena cavography is recommended. If collateral venous pathways are providing a bypass route around the filter or if thrombus is present above the existing filter, then a new suprarenal IVC filter may be placed.

Notes

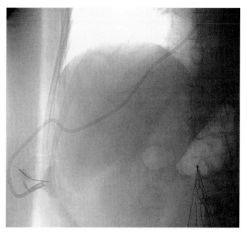

Courtesy of Dr. James Duncan.

1. What type of catheter is visualized?

2. What is the purpose of this procedure?

3. What vein has been accessed for this procedure?

4. If the jugular, subclavian, and femoral veins were occluded, what other route could be used to obtain central venous access?

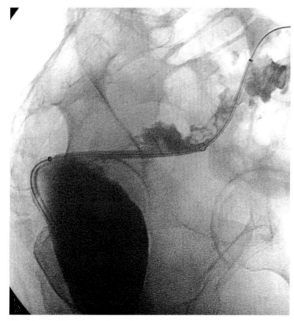

Courtesy of Dr. James Duncan.

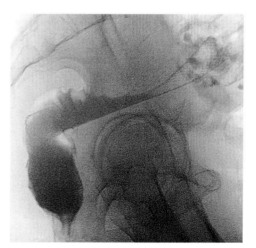

Courtesy of Dr. James Duncan.

1. What is the primary abnormality?

2. What procedure has been performed before the second image?

3. Would this be used in a patient with an anastomotic stricture?

4. Does this device need to be angioplastied during deployment?

CASE 160

Transhepatic Port Catheter Placement

1. Implantable port catheter.

2. To provide venous access.

3. Right hepatic vein.

4. Direct translumbar access into the inferior vena cava.

Reference

Johnson KL, Fellows KE, Murphy JD. Transhepatic central venous access for cardiac catheterization and radiologic intervention. *Cathet Cardiovasc Diagn.* 1995;35(2):168-171.

Cross-Reference

Vascular and Interventional Radiology: THE REQUISITES, pp 174-181.

Comment

Adults and children who undergo placement of multiple long-term central venous catheters are prone to develop chronic occlusions of these veins. After the jugular, subclavian, and femoral veins are all exhausted, limited options exist for further central venous access in these patients. When this occurs, a few approaches may be used: (1) Percutaneous recanalization of occluded central veins using angioplasty and/or stents might create enough of a channel through which a new long-term catheter can be placed; (2) Transhepatic venous access may be obtained as depicted here; (3) In extreme cases, translumbar access to the inferior vena cava may be obtained. Unfortunately, the first option may be extremely difficult or impossible, depending upon the chronicity of the occlusion. The last two options can usually be accomplished technically, but the catheter remains at some risk of migrating peripherally due to buckling outside the vein as the patient moves.

CASE 161

Colonic Stent Placement

1. Stricture at the rectosigmoid junction.

2. Colonic stent placement

3. No.

4. No.

Reference

Mergener K, Kozarik RA. Stenting of the gastrointestinal tract. *Dig Dis.* 2002;20(2):173-181.

Cross-Reference

Vascular and Interventional Radiology: THE REQUISITES, pp 543-555.

Comment

The images above depict placement of a large self-expanding Wallstent into the rectosigmoid colon, with subsequent relief of bowel obstruction.

Patients with malignant colorectal obstruction have historically required emergency laparotomy and two-stage bowel resection. In recent years, gastrointestinal tract stent placement has been used as a minimally invasive method of relieving large-bowel obstruction in two main subsets of patients. Those who present with acute symptoms may receive stent placement and then undergo treatment planning instead of high-risk emergency surgery. Patients with unresectable and metastatic disease might not require operation at all but might simply be treated palliatively by stent placement. This approach has the potential to spare patients the discomfort and morbidity of surgical bowel resection under inauspicious circumstances when quality of life should be the primary concern.

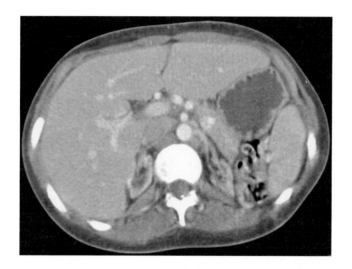

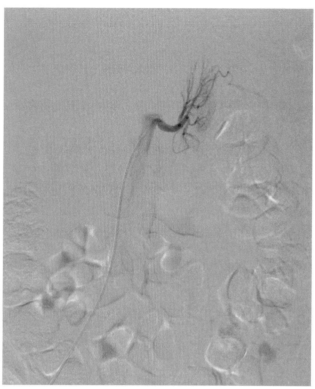

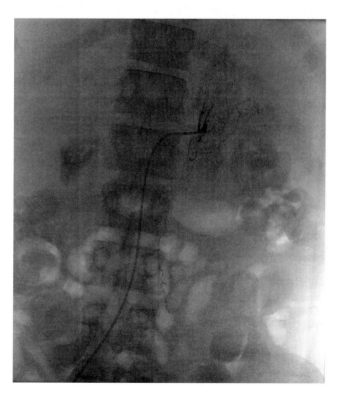

1. Describe the findings on the first image.

2. What procedure is being performed in the second image?

3. What procedure is being performed in the third image?

4. What are the indications for performing this procedure?

Renal Ablation for Hypertension

1. Bilateral atrophic kidneys.

2. Selective left renal arteriography.

3. Transarterial renal ablation.

4. Uncontrolled hypertension, nephritic syndrome, and autosomal dominant polycystic kidney disease.

References

Golwyn Jr DH, Routh WD, Chen MY, et al. Percutaneous transcatheter renal ablation with absolute ethanol for uncontrolled hypertension or nephrotic syndrome: Results in 11 patients with end-stage renal disease. *J Vasc Interv Radiol.* 1997;8:527-533.

Keller FS, Coyle M, Rosch J, et al. Percutaneous renal ablation in patients with end-stage renal disease: Alternative to surgical nephrectomy. *Radiology.* 1986;159:447-451.

Cross-Reference

Vascular and Interventional Radiology: THE REQUISITES, p 346.

Comment

Hypertension affects 80% of patients with end-stage renal disease and can sometimes be refractory to medical treatment. Surgical nephrectomy has been performed in the past in an attempt to treat uncontrolled hypertension in this patient population. Recently, transarterial renal ablation with absolute ethanol has been adopted by some centers as a less-invasive alternative therapy.

Ethanol in its concentrated form delivered selectively into the renal artery is cytotoxic and thrombogenic. Extreme care must be taken while infusing the ethanol to avoid reflux into the aorta. Infusion through a balloon-occlusion catheter may be performed to safeguard against this potentially devastating complication. The dilution effect that occurs once it traverses the renal parenchyma into the venous system renders it harmless, thus avoiding systemic complications.

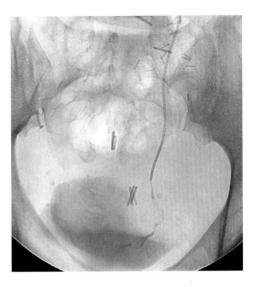
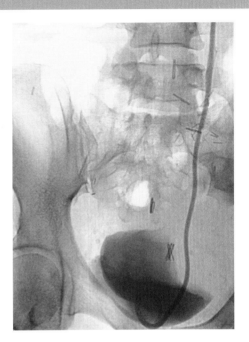

1. What study has been performed?

2. Name three imaging methods by which the ureter can be studied.

3. What is the primary finding in the first image?

4. What is the probable etiology of this finding?

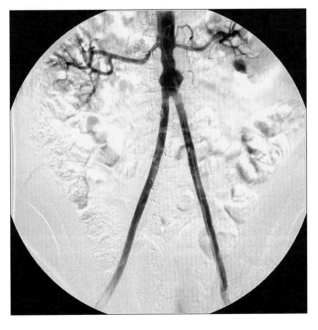
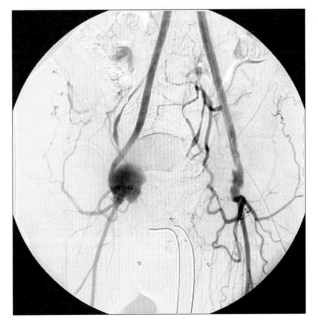

1. What surgical procedure has been performed?

2. What abnormality is present on the second image?

3. Name three methods of treating these vascular lesions.

4. Would stent-graft placement be good treatment for this abnormality?

CASE 163

Malignant Ureteral Stricture

1. Anterograde nephrostogram.

2. Anterograde pyelogram, retrograde pyelogram, intravenous pyelogram.

3. Tight irregular stricture of the distal left ureter.

4. Pelvic malignancy.

Reference

Blandino A, Gaeta M, Minutoli F, et al. MR urography of the ureter. *Am J Roentgenol.* 2002;179:1307-1314.

Cross-Reference

Vascular and Interventional Radiology: THE REQUISITES, pp 620-631.

Comment

The first image demonstrates a tight, irregular stricture of the left distal ureter. The imaging appearance strongly favors a malignant etiology for several reasons: the irregularity of the stricture; the presence of an irregular filling defect within the strictured segment, presumably representing tumor; and the presence of mass effect upon the ureter in the region of the stenosis and upon the adjacent bladder. However, in most instances pyelography alone will not be sufficient to determine the etiology of a ureteral stricture. In these cases, a knowledge of the patient's history and correlation with cross-sectional imaging modalities (to visualize a calculus, pelvic mass, or other lesion) may be helpful.

The treatment of malignant ureteral strictures depends largely upon the exact etiology and the overall extent of the disease. In many patients with bladder carcinoma and selected patients with other pelvic malignancies, total cystectomy with ileal conduit formation may be performed, obviating the need for percutaneous intervention. In many other patients, hydroureteronephrosis develops and is not likely to be relieved surgically. In these patients, percutaneous nephrostomy placement is usually performed, often followed by ureteral stent placement if bladder function is adequate. In the second image, the stenosis was successfully crossed and a nephroureteral stent was placed.

CASE 164

Femoral Anastomotic Pseudoaneurysm

1. Aortobifemoral bypass graft placement.

2. Right femoral anastomotic pseudoaneurysm.

3. Surgical repair, ultrasound-guided compression, percutaneous thrombin injection.

4. No. Stents and stent grafts should be avoided in the common femoral artery, because hip flexion can predispose to stent fracture.

References

Saad NE, Saad WE, Davies MG, et al. Pseudoaneurysms and the role of minimally invasive techniques in their management. *Radiographics.* 2005;25(Suppl 1): S173-S189.

Morgan R, Belli AM. Current treatment methods for postcatheterization pseudoaneurysms. *J Vasc Intervent Radiol.* 2003;14:697-710.

Cross-Reference

Vascular and Interventional Radiology: THE REQUISITES, p 436.

Comment

The development of an anastomotic pseudoaneurysm occurs in approximately 1% of patients per year after aortofemoral grafting. Anastomotic pseudoaneurysms are generally treated with surgical graft revision if the anastomosis is in a region that is readily amenable to surgical access. In carefully selected patients, a stent graft can be placed to address aortic pseudoaneurysms that arise near the proximal graft anastomosis. However, stent grafts are not used for femoral pseudoaneurysms.

Patients with postcatheterization femoral pseudoaneurysms may be treated by two relatively new percutaneous treatments. With ultrasound-guided compression therapy, the sonographer isolates the neck of the aneurysm and applies constant focal pressure to this region for 10 to 30 minutes; this form of therapy is effective in approximately 60% to 80% of cases; however, the recurrence rate after successful treatment may be as high as 20% to 30% in patients receiving anticoagulant therapy. For these reasons, ultrasound-guided compression of the pseudoaneurysm neck has largely been replaced with direct percutaneous injection of thrombin into the sac, which produces instant pseudoaneurysm thrombosis. This technique is faster and more effective (>90% of patients) than ultrasound-guided compression therapy. Surgical treatment is needed for several groups of patients: those with infected or rapidly expanding pseudoaneurysms; those with distal ischemia or neuropathy caused by local pressure by the pseudoaneurysm upon the femoral artery or nerve, respectively; and those who fail percutaneous management.

CASE 165

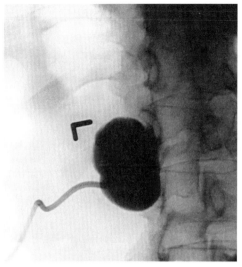

Courtesy of Dr. Michael Darcy.

1. Name three renal fluid collections for which percutaneous nephrostomy access might be needed.

2. In what situations are uninfected renal cysts drained percutaneously?

3. What therapy can be employed to treat symptomatic renal cysts that do not respond to simple aspiration?

4. Do patients undergoing renal cyst drainage tend to require long-term drainage?

CASE 166

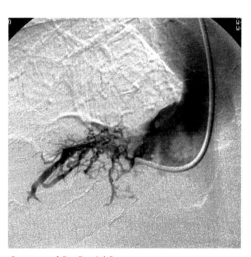 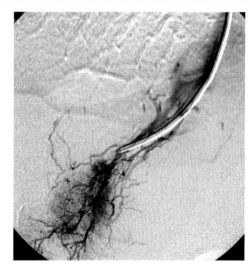

Courtesy of Dr. Daniel Brown.　　　　*Courtesy of Dr. Daniel Brown.*

1. What veins have been selected in the images shown?

2. What vessels are opacified?

3. What is the diagnosis?

4. What test is the gold standard for diagnosis of this problem?

Renal Cyst Sclerosis

1. Renal abscess (for drainage), stone-containing calyceal diverticulum (to facilitate percutaneous stone removal), and symptomatic renal cyst (for sclerosis).

2. Chronic pain, recurrence after needle aspiration.

3. Ethanol sclerosis.

4. No.

Reference

Paananen I, Hellstrom P, Leinonen S, et al. Treatment of renal cysts with single-session percutaneous drainage and ethanol sclerotherapy: Long-term outcome. *Urology.* 2001;57:30-33.

Cross-Reference

Vascular and Interventional Radiology: THE REQUISITES, pp 509-510.

Comment

The vast majority of simple renal cysts do not require any form of treatment. However, a small number of patients do complain of significant pain associated with the presence of a large, dominant cyst. In these patients, several percutaneous treatment methods can be used. Renal cyst aspiration via a needle may be performed; many patients respond to this limited form of therapy, although in a large percentage symptoms recur. For this reason, ethanol ablation therapy can be performed either as the first approach or after a trial of aspiration has failed.

Under ultrasound and fluoroscopic guidance, a needle is positioned in the cyst, and a drainage catheter is placed over a guidewire. The cyst is aspirated dry. Contrast is injected into the cyst to ensure that no communication is present with the renal collecting system and to define the volume of the cyst. The contrast is aspirated and is replaced with a smaller volume of absolute ethanol. Protocols vary, but in general the ethanol is allowed to dwell for 15 minutes as the patient periodically changes position. The contrast is then aspirated. This procedure may be repeated twice at the initial sitting. The catheter is then left to gravity drainage.

Budd–Chiari Syndrome

1. Accessory right hepatic vein and main right hepatic vein.

2. Hepatic venous collaterals.

3. Budd–Chiari syndrome (BCS).

4. Hepatic venography.

Reference

Mancuso A, Fung K, Mela M, et al. TIPS for acute and chronic Budd–Chiari syndrome: A single-centre experience. *J Hepatol.* 2003;38(6):751-754.

Cross-Reference

Vascular and Interventional Radiology: THE REQUISITES, pp 399-401.

Comment

Patients with BCS present with severe ascites (85%-90% of patients), hepatosplenomegaly, abdominal pain, jaundice, vomiting, and/or extremity edema. If untreated, BCS patients develop progressive portal hypertension with esophageal variceal bleeding, encephalopathy, hepatic failure, and death. BCS can be caused by tumor invasion of the inferior vena cava (IVC) or hepatic veins, membranous suprahepatic IVC obstruction, right atrial tumors, polycythemia vera, postpartum state, oral contraceptive use, paroxysmal nocturnal hemoglobinuria, veno-occlusive disease (in patients who have received chemotherapy and radiation), and various hematologic conditions.

CT and MRI findings in BCS include hepatomegaly, ascites, inhomogeneous hepatic enhancement with a fan-shaped area of decreasing peripheral enhancement, and caudate lobe enlargement. Duplex ultrasound can demonstrate hepatic vein flow to be absent, reversed, turbulent, or monophasic. Hepatic venography, the gold standard for diagnosis, can demonstrate webs, stenosis, or thrombus within the suprahepatic IVC or hepatic veins with abundant collaterals (well depicted above) between the main hepatic veins.

Patients with BCS due to IVC or hepatic vein stenosis may be treated effectively with balloon angioplasty or stent placement (when stenosis recurs following angioplasty). Patients with IVC thrombosis may be treated with thrombolytic therapy. Patients with hepatic vein thrombosis have been successfully treated with TIPS, although this may be technically difficult to perform and the long-term results of this approach are unknown.

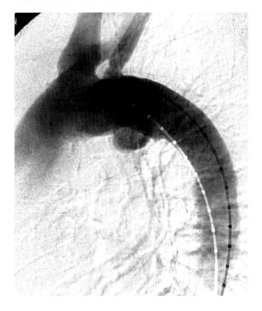 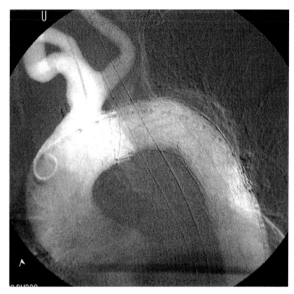

1. What abnormality is seen in the first image?

2. How has this been treated?

3. What may have happened to the left subclavian artery?

4. Are thoracic aortic stent grafts also prone to endoleaks and migration over time?

Thoracic Aortic Stent-Graft Placement

1. Thoracic aortic aneurysm along the underside of the distal part of the aortic arch.

2. Stent-graft placement.

3. It was probably ligated surgically before stent-graft placement.

4. Yes.

Reference

Sakai T, Dake MD, Semba CP, et al. Descending thoracic aortic aneurysm: Thoracic CT findings after endovascular stent-graft placement. *Radiology*. 1999;212:169-174.

Cross-Reference

Vascular and Interventional Radiology: THE REQUISITES, pp 233-235.

Comment

Surgical repair of thoracic aortic aneurysms is associated with the complications of death in 6% to 12%, paraplegia in 3% to 16%, and cardiorespiratory problems in 20% to 30%. Stent-graft repair has hence been viewed as a welcome treatment alternative.

Like abdominal aortic aneurysms, the status of the proximal and distal aneurysm necks (which must be >2 cm length and free of significant angulation and plaque) and of the iliac arteries (which must be >7-8 mm) are important factors in determining eligibility for endovascular thoracic aortic aneurysm repair. Other considerations specific to the thoracic aorta include: (1) The degree of thoracic aortic curvature; (2) The relationship of the aneurysm to the left subclavian artery: if a 2-cm proximal neck is not present, then the subclavian artery may first be surgically ligated (as in this case); alternatively, it may be covered with the stent graft, provided there is a good seal to prevent a type II endoleak. (Patients with a dominant left vertebral artery, an incomplete vertebrobasilar system, or a left internal mammary artery to coronary artery bypass graft should undergo revascularization before the origin of the left subclavian artery is covered); (3) The location of key intercostal arteries: Although no definite relationship to paraplegia has been established, it is wise to minimize coverage of patent intercostal arteries.

The large initial experience with stent grafts for TAA has mostly used homemade devices, in which a stent was sutured to graft material by the operator. Using these rudimentary devices, initial aneurysm exclusion rates have been 80% to 100%. However, at 4-year follow-up, only about 50% are free of endoleak.

Notes

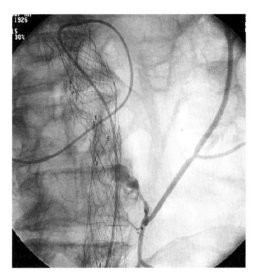

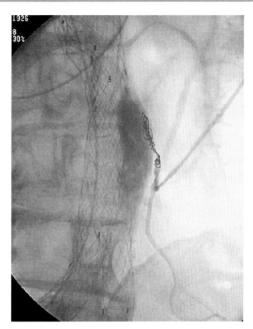

Courtesy of Dr. David Hovsepian.

Courtesy of Dr. David Hovsepian.

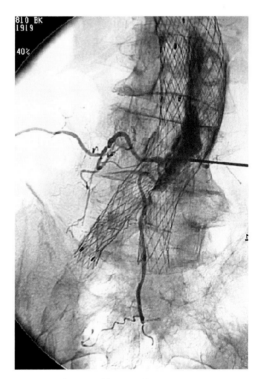

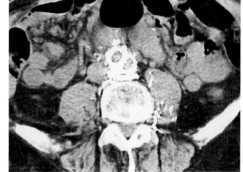

Courtesy of Dr. David Hovsepian.

Courtesy of Dr. David Hovsepian.

1. What diagnosis do Patient A (top two images) and Patient B (bottom two images) have in common?

2. In Patient A, what vascular circuits supply the abnormality?

3. Is this abnormality related to poor initial device positioning?

4. On the CT scan of Patient B (last image), what is the hyperattenuating material posterior to the stent graft?

Embolization of Type II Endoleak

1. Type II endoleak after endoluminal grafting.

2. Superior mesenteric artery, middle colic artery, marginal artery, inferior mesenteric artery, endoleak.

3. No.

4. Embolization glue that has been injected directly into the aneurysm sac, filling the nearby patent lumbar arteries.

Reference

Kasirajan K, Matteson B, Marek JM, et al. Technique and results of transfemoral superselective coil embolization of type II lumbar endoleak. *J Vasc Surg*. 2003; 38:61-66.

Cross-Reference

Vascular and Interventional Radiology: THE REQUISITES, pp 256-260.

Comment

The top left image demonstrates a type II endoleak due to retrograde flow in the inferior mesenteric artery. The top right image demonstrates successful placement of embolization coils in the feeding branch, which resulted in closure of the endoleak. When the feeding vessel can be catheterized, this provides an effective treatment method.

The bottom left image demonstrates a type II endoleak due to retrograde flow in lumbar arteries. The bottom left image depicts filling of the aneurysm sac and the patent lumbar arteries via direct translumbar puncture of the aneurysm sac. The CT scan on the bottom right demonstrates injected *N*-bucrylate glue posterior to the stent-graft device and within the aneurysm sac and lumbar branches. Early aneurysm thrombosis has been observed following direct injection of glue or thrombin into the aneurysm sac, and this option may be particularly useful in patients in whom catheterization of the feeding artery is difficult. However, the long-term results of this approach (and of coil embolization) in producing durable aneurysm exclusion are unknown.

Notes

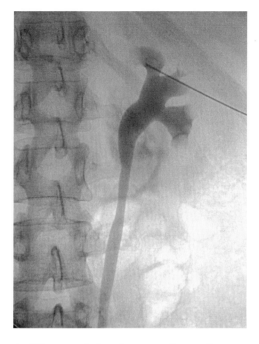
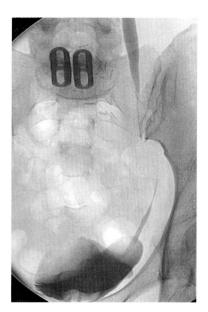

1. What study has been performed?

2. What abnormality is seen?

3. Name two noninvasive tests that could be used to determine if the visualized abnormality is causing functional obstruction.

4. Name one invasive test that could be used to determine if the visualized abnormality is causing functional obstruction.

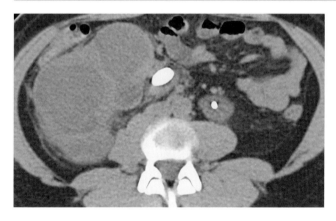

1. What is the diagnosis on this noncontrast CT scan?

2. If the patient is afebrile, why would percutaneous nephrostomy be performed?

3. When percutaneous stone removal is being performed, what calyx usually provides the easiest access into the ureter?

4. Name two potential complications that can result from use of this calyx.

CASE 169

Whitaker Test

1. Anterograde pyelogram.

2. Ureteral stricture.

3. Intravenous pyelogram, diuretic renal scintigraphy.

4. Whitaker test.

Reference

Tchetgen MB, Bloom DA. Robert H. Whitaker and the Whitaker test: A pressure-flow study of the upper urinary tract. *Urology*. 2003;61:253-256.

Cross-Reference

Vascular and Interventional Radiology: THE REQUISITES, pp 606-607.

Comment

The images demonstrate an anterograde pyogram in which a stenosis is present in the distal ureter. In this patient with repeated upper urinary tract infections, diuretic scintigraphy was equivocal as to whether true obstruction was present. For this reason, a Whitaker test was performed and was negative. If the test had been positive, a percutaneous nephrostomy catheter and/or ureteral stent would have been left in place.

To perform a Whitaker test, catheterization of the bladder and needle placement in the renal pelvis is performed. During infusion of dilute contrast at a fixed rate (10 mL/min for 9 minutes, then 15 mL/min for 9 minutes is one commonly used protocol), manometry of the bladder (to estimate resting intraabdominal pressure) and renal pelvis is performed every 3 minutes. The true renal pelvis pressure is calculated as the difference between these two pressures at each time interval. If the pressures reach 22 cm H_2O, then the test is clearly positive; if the pressures stay below 15 cm H_2O, then the test is clearly negative. Reproduction of flank pain symptoms with pressures in the borderline zone is also considered by most physicians to represent a positive test.

CASE 170

Ureteral Calculus

1. Right hydronephrosis with right ureteral calculus.

2. To preserve renal function, to facilitate percutaneous stone removal.

3. Upper-pole calyx.

4. Traversal of the pleural space can cause pneumothorax or urothorax.

Reference

Landman J, Venkatesh R, Lee DI, et al. Combined percutaneous and retrograde approach to staghorn calculi with application of the ureteral access sheath to facilitate percutaneous nephrolithotomy. *J Urol*. 2003; 169:64-67.

Cross-Reference

Vascular and Interventional Radiology: THE REQUISITES, pp 615-619.

Comment

The noncontrast CT images demonstrate a large calculus at the right ureteropelvic junction. The kidney is hydronephrotic and shows marked parenchymal thinning suggesting long-term chronic obstruction. Urgent percutaneous nephrostomy tube placement is indicated if the patient is febrile. If the patient shows no signs of infection, then percutaneous nephrostomy can be electively performed to preserve renal function and/or to facilitate percutaneous stone removal. Evaluation for the presence of significant residual function in the right kidney via renal scintigraphy would be advised before placing a nephrostomy tube in that kidney.

To perform percutaneous stone removal, obtaining optimal access into the renal collecting system is extremely important. Typically the collecting system is accessed and a guidewire is passed into the bladder and snared from below to obtain through-and-through access. A balloon catheter is then used to dilate the subcutaneous tract to accommodate a large (often 30 F) sheath. Through this sheath, a nephroscope is passed into the renal collecting system, and under direct visualization the stone is fragmented and removed. A nephrostomy catheter, and sometimes a ureteral stent, is left in place after the procedure.

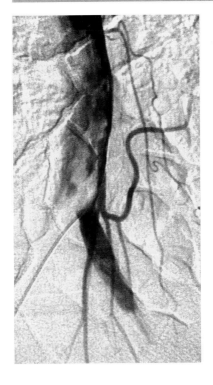
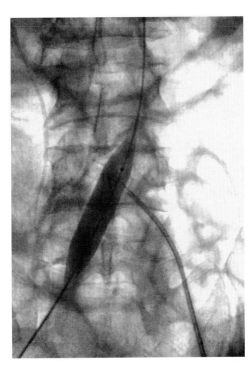
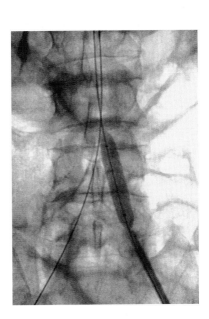
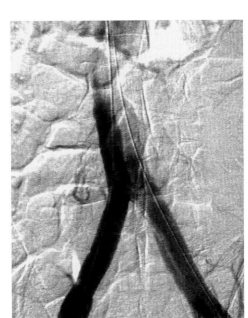

1. From where do the left common iliac artery and inferior mesenteric artery derive their blood supply in this patient?

2. What procedure is being performed in the remaining images?

3. Why is this procedure performed?

4. What is the purpose of the angioplasty balloon in the second image?

Percutaneous Balloon Fenestration of Aortic Dissection

1. From the collapsed true lumen of a dissected aorta.

2. Percutaneous balloon fenestration of the intimal flap.

3. Lower-limb ischemia in the setting of acute aortic dissection.

4. To serve as a fluoroscopically visible target for transseptal needle puncture.

Reference

Slonim SM, Miller DC, Mitchell RS, et al. Percutaneous balloon fenestration and stenting for life-threatening ischemia complications in patients with acute aortic dissection. *J Thorac Cardiovasc Surg*. 1999;117: 1118-1127.

Cross-Reference

Vascular and Interventional Radiology: THE REQUI-SITES, pp 235-239.

Comment

The first image demonstrates a pelvic angiogram in a patient with acute type B aortic dissection and left leg ischemia. A collapsed true lumen supplies the inferior mesenteric and left common iliac arteries. The second image demonstrates placement of a target balloon in the aortic false lumen from the right iliac artery, and guided puncture of the balloon using a needle from the left iliac artery true lumen. The third image shows transseptal flap angioplasty, and the final image demonstrates flow from the false lumen crossing the newly created aortic fenestration to supply the left common iliac artery. This patient's ischemic symptoms resolved instantly and he did not require surgery.

Patients with acute type B dissection complicated by visceral or peripheral arterial ischemia are at high risk for death and paraplegia during surgical aortic repair. For this reason, several percutaneous methods have been used to relieve organ ischemia in these patients. Stents can be placed in branch vessels that are dissected. In addition, patients with true lumen collapse and organ ischemia due to poor inflow to a true lumen-supplied branch artery can be treated with percutaneous balloon fenestration (shown here) or aortic stent placement; in early studies, perfusion was successfully restored to tissue beds that were more than 90% ischemic using these methods. Another endovascular approach involves placement of a stent graft across the primary intimal dissection tear in the thoracic aorta.

Notes